beauty bible
beauty steals

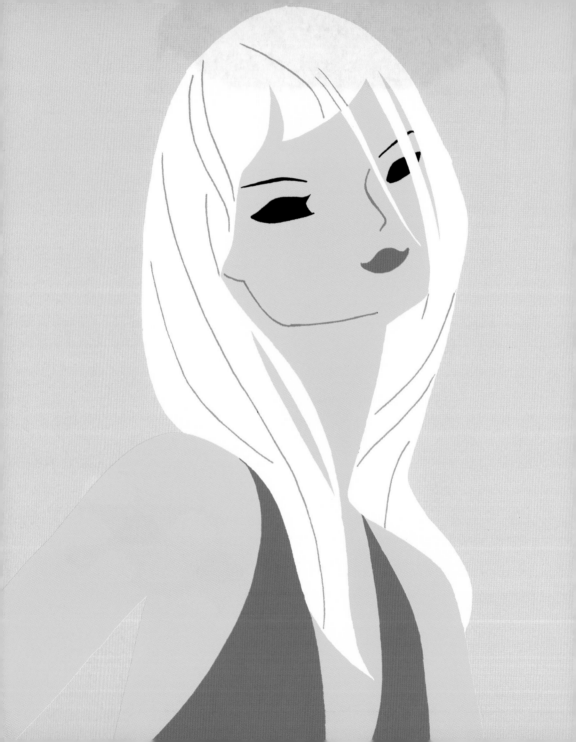

beauty bible
beauty steals

by Sarah Stacey and Josephine Fairley

with illustrations by
Orlando Hoetzel

Kyle Cathie Limited

contents

Dear Beauty Bible beauty-hound,

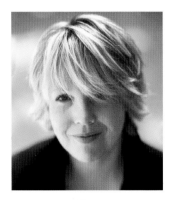

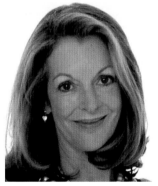

Our mission has always been to help you save time and money, with a fast-track to products that really work. And actually, long before the global financial meltdown forced us all to question what we spend, we knew that you don't have to spend a fortune to find great beauty buys, right across the product spectrum.

Since we started writing the Beauty Bible series, we've always flagged up the Beauty Steals in every Tried & Tested category. Then, well before credit really got crunched, Jo's bags got lost on the way to a family wedding in the American Midwest. Forced to restock her make-up bag via the shelves of Wal-Mart at Lake Okoboji (we kid you not), she went on a supermarket sweep of brands like L'Oréal, Rimmel, Revlon and Max Factor, and was reminded that there are truly stupendous products available for very little money indeed. And many have held pride of place in Jo's kit, long since she was reunited with her more costly lotions, potions, creams and powders.

So, the winning products that appear in this book cost little. Virtually nothing over £10 – except for some miracle creams, eye treatments and cellulite-blitzers where we felt that £20 wasn't too steep for a true miracle. (And, there really are budget anti-ageing miracle workers.) And when you see a product marked SuperSteal, it means it's under a fiver – pretty unbelievable, until you read all the testers' reports.

Every product we trial – and there are hundreds, across 67 categories, from make-up to suncare, via hair, body and anti-ageing – goes to panels of ten real women, living in real-world conditions, who then fill in intensive questionnaires. With key categories, we ask our testers to trial them on one side only, for comparison. Differences soon became apparent with the really effective products, triggering the usual flurry of requests from testers who want to start using said product on the other side – because the changes become visible not just to our doughty testers, but to husbands, colleagues, friends…

Please, keep this book by your side when you shop, because there is an awful lot of mediocre skincare, haircare and bodycare (and make-up) on the high street. The products that made it to the pages of this book got good marks, and performed well. But plenty of others got derisory scores. Spending a fiver on a product that doesn't perform may not break the bank – but it's still £5 more than anyone has to waste.

The downside of shopping for make-up and skincare in a supermarket or a high-street drugstore (let alone over the internet) is that there are no tester units, and no beauty consultants. And who has time to scrutinise every ingredient list, or fathom the differences between suncare that's identically packaged, but might be anything from a self-tanner to a high-SPF sun cream? We went half-crazed trying to unravel some packaging – and that was with the help of a magnifying glass and a personal hotline to the relevant brand's PR office.

So, think of *Beauty Steals* as your portable beauty consultant; what's more, one who'll give it to you straight – because we're totally, completely, 100 per cent independent.

Also, we hope you'll enjoy some of the best money-saving beauty secrets we've ever learned: ways to extend the time between your salon treatments; how to blag beauty freebies; products that do double duty, and lots of others.

So, the bottom line is: why pay more?

www.beautybible.com

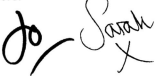

What the symbols mean

The products in this book are all 'beauty steals', most costing under £10 sterling. In a very few cases (eg. miracle creams), we have upped the £10 ceiling, but never to more than £20.

 Lots of products are SuperSteals, which means they cost under £5 sterling; they are marked 'SuperSteal', inside a purse!

Some products have one to three daisies by their name. This refers to their content of natural ingredients:

❀ ONE DAISY is for products that are principally botanical and/or mineral, with a small percentage of synthetic or petrochemical ingredients.

❀❀ TWO DAISIES, as above, but with no synthetic or petrochemical ingredients.

❀❀❀ THREE DAISIES means the product is certified organic by one of the leading organic certifiers.

your beauty tool kit

Using the right brushes can make cheapo cosmetics look a million dollars. Make-up artist Jenny Jordan trialled a huge range of budget brushes for us at her North London Eyebrow and Make-up Clinic. These are the ones she rates as top value – soft, don't moult, well shaped for the job and will last well.

Remember: the trick with application is blend, blend, blend…

Foundation brush: No 7 Foundation Brush
Jenny says: 'This has lots of softness and body, didn't moult at all and is very well shaped. It worked really well with both liquid foundation and dry mineral powder – both glided on, and the shape allowed you to take it right up to the lash line. It's just over the £10 mark, but really worth it.'

Powder brush: EcoTools Powder Brush
Jenny says: 'This has a beautifully domed shape, and although the hairs are light and loose, it holds the powder well. It feels dreamily soft, unlike other ones, which were a bit scratchy. By far the most luxurious.' (Also available in a good-value set.)

Blush brush: Avon Blusher Brush
Jenny says: 'Angled brushes are great for application, as they wrap the colour round your cheekbones but you don't get too much. Brush up and out, with the short side on your cheekbones. This is not the softest ever, but the cut makes up for it.'

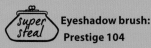 **Eyeshadow brush: Prestige 104 Shadow Sweep**
Jenny says: 'Forget those little sponge applicators that come with eyeshadow: using a brush with a soft, flat nib to blend eyeshadow all over your eyelids makes a big difference. This looks and feels really expensive.'

Eye contour brush: Revlon Contour Shadow Brush
Jenny says: 'Dip the tip into your eye shadow, then draw it back and forth in the socket for ages to give a 3D effect. This brush is soft, really well shaped and effective.'

tip Tweezers are another vital tool. We prefer a slant-ended version (rather than pointed or rounded) and would rather invest more in award-winning Tweezerman Pink Slant tweezers than fumble around with cheap versions.

tip

Cotton-wool buds (and pads) are vital accessories for all manner of beauty chores, including dipping into eye make-up remover to take off any errant splodges under your eyes – although, for that, you could always try Smudgees Eye Make-Up Smudge Removers – 20 individually wrapped mini-wands, all for under a fiver. Small objects of genius!

 super steal **Lip brush: Elegant Touch Lip Brush**

Jenny says: 'A real bargain. Although not retractable, it has a cover, which is great for travelling: just put some lippy on the end, and that's all you need to take. Good shape for outlining and filling in, but top up with lip gloss to make your mouth look sexy/pouty.'

Concealer brush:
Jenny says: 'Buy a tiny fine paint brush from any art store; dip into concealer and dab on to the blemish, or push into frown lines. Use it for eyeliner, too, to get really close to the lash line.'

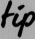 ## tip

Wash old mascara brushes and use them to separate lashes, and to brush eyebrows.

tried & tested
anti-ageing
eye creams

Tackling fine lines and wrinkles in the eye zone is one of beauty's biggest challenges. So it was a real eye-opener to find that, even if several do slightly exceed our £10 price ceiling, these inexpensive age-defying eye products outscored brands charging ten times as much.

Liz Earle Naturally Active Skincare Daily Eye Repair

7.68/10 We always feel that Liz Earle's products deliver great value – here, an intensive cream containing concentrated botanicals including echinacea, light-reflective pigments and a useful SPF10.

Testers say: 'Amazed to see a visible difference: the eye I used this on was so much better, with finer lines' • 'instantly blurred lines; worked very well on puffiness; camouflaged dark circles' • 'sank in quickly' • 'good base for concealer' • 'should be marketed as an eye and lip treatment: noticeable improvement in both areas – lifting and firming'.

L'Oréal Age Re-Perfect Pro-Calcium De-Crinkling Eye & Lip Contours

7.4/10 Wow: the first of three L'Oréal products in this category. Pro-Calcium is a stable form of calcium which can be absorbed by the skin, improving barrier function, L'Oréal claim. A tad over a tenner.

Testers say: 'Wrinkles much less prominent, fine lines seemed to disappear; eyes looked bright, dark circles less dark, puffiness reduced' • 'people say I look less tired' • 'I think this is best suited for very mature skin' • 'I was sceptical but it was good for me: lessening of dark circles, made under-eye skin feel and look stronger'.

L'Oréal Wrinkle De-Crease Collagen Filler Eye

7.4/10 We asked testers to trial this in the short term as a 'line-filler' (and it did well, see page 77). But it rose even better to the challenge of delivering longer-term improvements. With regular use, L'Oréal say the eye contour area will look 'plumper, softer and visibly rejuvenated'.

Testers say: 'A wondrous effect on brightening my eye area; my dark circles almost removed; and brilliantly hydrating too' • 'the instant sheen made skin look fresh, and lines less' • 'perfect consistency; sank in immediately' • 'I didn't expect miracles but I did get effectiveness: lovely!'.

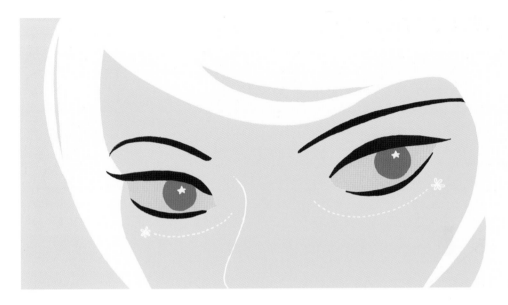

Nivea Visage Expert Lift Eye Cream

7.39/10 The Expert Lift range targets women from 50-65, incorporating 'Bioxilift': a '100 per cent natural' ingredient derived from the anise plant, said to boost collagen activity, together with hyaluronic acid.

Testers say: 'Lovely consistency; absorbed very quickly and felt hydrating; lines a bit smoother and finer, eyes brighter, puffiness reduced, definite effect on my dark circles'•'slightly blurred the wrinkles when I applied it'•'with continued use this lessened the number and length of crow's feet. Honestly! I went from three long ones to two short ones'.

Yes to Carrots Eye Can See Clearly Now Eye Contour Cream

7/10 The least expensive of the eye products that did well in this trial, featuring anti-inflammatory green tea, plus smoothing aloe vera and the brand's mega-antioxidant blend.

Testers say: 'I loved it! The cream looked like Angel Delight; sank in easily, skin felt nicely hydrated and lines maybe slightly softer'• 'more hydrating than my normal product, competitively priced, moisturised beautifully, and lines were smoother'•'decent size pot! Really worked: eyes brighter, wrinkles less prominent, puffiness reduced'.

L'Oréal Derma-Genesis Cellular-Youth Nurturing Eye Contour Cream

7/10 This silky lightweight product is light-reflective – so there's an instant 'cosmetic' benefit, with under-eye dark circles reduced. Key anti-ager is Pro-Xylane™, which 'plumps, tautens, illuminates, brightens'.

Testers say: 'I liked the feel of this, and it does the job expected! Skin looks smoother, make-up glides on, the eye area looks younger'•'reduced puffiness'• 'improvement in fine lines after six weeks, wrinkles less defined, whole eye area looked lifted and more youthful, dark circles improved – I was delighted'

tried & tested
miracle creams

Our ultimate Beauty Bible challenge is identifying creams that deliver actual, visible, commented-on-by-others improvements to skin, helping to turn back the ageing clock. And we've always known that, amazingly, the results delivered by affordable creams rival those of infinitely more expensive options.

For this category we set a higher 'ceiling' of £20 – mainly because, as we've noted elsewhere in this book, the minute the promise of 'anti-ageing' is linked to a skincare product, prices tend to be higher. We know this is partly a reflection of companies having to recoup huge research and development budgets, but we also have an inkling that it taps into women's anxieties about the ageing process, and their willingness to do (and spend) almost anything to stop it in its tracks (which, of course, brands know very well). But in this age of the £1,500 anti-ageing product – yikes! – these are true bargains.

L'Oréal Derma-Genesis Cellular-Youth Nurturing Night Cream

8.3/10 We trialled more than 60 anti-ageing 'beauty steals' for this category from dozens of brands – yet three out of the top nine highest-scoring products spring from L'Oréal's labs (including the Garnier products): a result which reflects their huge commitment to age-defying R & D. This is the night product from the same range which scored well in our anti-ageing eye treatment Tried & Tested: it also contains high levels of skin-plumping hyaluronic acid, plus L'Oréal's patented Pro-Xylane™ ingredient. (NB: one tester linked a sensitivity reaction to this.)

Testers say: 'Gorgeous product; lavender-coloured light cream which is quickly absorbed and a real pleasure to use; the first morning my skin was brighter and slightly plumped; after two weeks, fine lines across forehead and round mouth less visible; neck smoothed, and complexion dramatically brightened – people have commented!'•'delighted to find such an effective product at a price I could afford'•'nourishing and relaxing'•'skin was smoother and plumper'•'after a few weeks, dry areas did not need extra moisturiser'•'definite reduction in wrinkles; more even skin tone'.

Neal's Yard Remedies Frankincense Nourishing Cream ❀

8.25/10 This has long appeared in other books of ours, but we re-tested it – and again, it got spectacular results (though a few testers found it heavy). The rich botanical cream, the most natural in this section, has high levels of frankincense essential oil, used in mummification – so no wonder it's so good at preserving skin. The blend includes oils of wheatgerm, almond and myrrh, renowned for regenerating and moisturising properties. It can be applied at night and also under make-up.

Testers say: 'I thought it would be too rich for my oily skin but it was miraculous! Skin looked so much younger and plumper, and it seemed to reduce breakouts – my skin tone changed: I've never seen such initial dramatic effects maintained' • 'immediate feeling of plumpness has been replaced by a smooth uplift and youthful tightness, yet skin feels comfortable' • 'I always felt my skin looked colourless and grey until I tested this' • after two weeks I went out without foundation, which I've never done before' • 'no adverse reactions on my sensitive skin' • 'noticeable improvement in brightness and translucency' • 'healthy and "strong" feeling to my skin now' • 'a real winter cream you feel is protecting you' • 'spots clear quicker; old scarring improved'.

Soap & Glory Make Yourself Youthful Rejuvenating Face Serum

8.12/10 A triumph for Marcia Kilgore with this light, sinks-in-fast serum. It is probably all oily skins need (under 50), but can be layered under something richer for dry skins. It contains a collagen-stimulating tetrapeptide, an 'organic oxygenating complex', ginseng, shea butter, sweet orange peel essential oil and a 'moisture-trapping complex'.

Testers say: 'Glided on the skin wonderfully and sank in quickly; I used as a serum with a moisturiser on top, morning and night – after two weeks, a marked improvement in skin tone and softness, fine lines less evident, skin had a lovely bright glow – my son commented! Wonderful!' • 'pleasant orange aroma; significant improvement in radiance in first 24 hours, skin on neck and chest smoother, less crepey, more hydrated; fine lines a little softer' • 'a great serum at a very good price'.

Nivea Visage DNAge Cell Renewal Night Cream

 7.55/10 You might think from this name that Nivea has harnessed the power of human DNA in a skin cream – but actually, it simply contains creatine and folic acid, to protect skin cells (and therefore DNA) from damage. Targeted at women from 40 to 55, this patent-pending product focuses on the key challenges facing that age group – in particular, loss of elasticity and firmness. NB: one tester did experience a sensitivity reaction, which brought the average down.

Testers say: 'After two weeks, fine lines smoother and wrinkles not as deep, skin healthier and plumper; very noticeable difference between the side I used it on and the other' • 'absorbed very quickly with no residue' • 'skin looked lovely and clear and definitely brighter and smoother, as if I'd had a good night's sleep – which unfortunately I hadn't' • 'my nose-to-mouth groove was greatly improved' • 'definite improvement in brightness – really liked the rich creamy texture; you only need a small amount' • 'I wake up now with hydrated soft skin even after a late night' • 'will definitely buy'.

♡ we love

Jo's a long, long-term fan of Neal's Yard Remedies Frankincense Nourishing Cream (*left*). Sarah plumps for Essential Care products, particularly Organic Rose Moisturiser and Avocado Replenishing Cream.

Healthspan Nurture Replenish Collagen Boosting Serum

 7.35/10 The Replenish line (from this mail-order-only skincare and supplements company), targeted at 50-plus women, contains plant oestrogens from soybean extract, plus Matryxyl 3000 and RonaCareVTA, to help inhibit collagen degradation. The light, very smooth-feeling serum comes in an airless pump.

Testers say: 'Light lotion, easy to apply and fairly quick to absorb; skin immediately softer and smoother – even dry areas; complexion is brighter, more even in tone and texture'•'slight reduction in fine lines around eyes; skin generally less tired looking'• skin on neck improved too'•'definite improvement in brightness'•'skin was so smooth that make-up went on beautifully and stayed put all day. My partner says my skin feels like silk'.

Pond's Regener-Activ Deep Night Treatment

 super steal

7.3/10 All products in Pond's Regener-Activ range contain marine collagen and pro-retinol microcapsules, supposed to stimulate the natural generation process. This was the cheapest of the anti-ageing products that did well, so, although it's a little bit over a fiver, it's our SuperSteal.

Testers say: 'Very light, fluffy cream which melted into my skin; next morning my skin was glowing, soft, smooth and lighter and brighter, with fine lines plumped and more even skin tone'•'if you look brighter, as I do, you look refreshed and therefore younger'•'my dry skin lapped up this cream, and felt smoother and silkier'•'lines around lips and eyes improved, slightly improved bigger wrinkles'•'fine lines reduced'•'love the texture and the way it sinks in'.

Garnier UltraLift Pro-X Re-plumping Day Cream

 7.28/10 The first of two Garnier products which scored very similar marks: the UltraLift Pro-X features Pro-Xylane®, derived from beech trees, to help plump, firm and smooth skin. This option does not have an SPF, so if you really want to protect against ageing you'd need to layer one over or under.

Testers say: 'Rich, silky texture; good for ageing dry skin; leaves a slight sheen and a bit of a glow; kept skin moisturised and plump'•'after two weeks, skin looks different – improvement in softness, crepiness and fine lines'•'fine lines reduced around the treated eye'•'wonderful unscented creamy texture that goes a long way and sinks in very quickly; fine lines less noticeable, bigger wrinkles softer: brighter, smoother, younger-looking skin'.

Garnier UltraLift Pro-X Intensive Night Replumping & Anti-Wrinkle Regenerating Night Cream

7.17/10 This new addition to the Pro-X range is the night-time counterpart of the Day Cream (*above*) which just pipped it to the post, score-wise. It harnesses the same anti-ageing molecules (Pro-Xylane®), but is

tip **'The secret to eternal youth: wear sunscreen, even on cloudy days. (Don't forget your neck and hands.) While people perceive tanned skin to look healthy, it is a sign that your skin is screaming. UV rays leave you with DNA damage, which gives you age spots and leads to "sag". My middle name is "anti-tan". Just fake it!'** *Marcia Kilgore* applied at night, when skin regeneration is at its peak. L'Oreal tell us 'skin will feel more toned and plumper'. Among our testers, there were raves, one sensitivity reaction, and a couple couldn't get on with the smell.

Testers say: 'Ten out of ten! Skin is silky smooth and soft, slightly plumper' • 'lovely texture; skin feels much smoother and brighter; neck feels like it's less old' • 'I actually like looking at myself now; my hairdresser commented on skin softness compared to others my age' • 'I'm prone to redness but nowhere as bad now, and no dry flakiness' • 'a plumping effect which does wonders! Lovely protecting, moisturising properties' • 'this rich thick cream, based on mineral oil, feels great on my skin' • 'fine lines on forehead seem less definite' • 'fairly rich cream, sank into skin easily; skin did look brighter and more radiant, though slightly taut feeling for first few days – needed facial oil as well for my dry skin'.

Dr Nick Lowe Night Recovery Cream

7.11/10 Dr Nick Lowe is a skin guru beloved of beauty editors: he's someone we all turn to for sage advice. Now he's brought out his own range – and

The neck's best thing

While the anti-ageing face creams we tried did amazingly well, rivalling more expensive brands, the budget neck creams performed poorly in general – and the only one that did creditably has been discontinued! So we have a suggestion: simply extend your anti-aging face cream down your neck and décolletage – NB: we always suggest stroking a product up to your jawline from your bosom, alternating both sets of fingertips in a sweeping movement and being careful to include all of your bosom and all round the neck.

In fact, one of our favourite anti-ageing creams, **Skin Repair Moisturiser by Liz Earle Naturally Active Skincare**, scored highly when submitted as a neck cream in *The Green Beauty Bible*, gaining **7.85/10**. The full size comes in at over our £10 ceiling, but you can buy a trial size for much less – and using one product for face and neck will save pennies, of course. Ingredients include echinacea, borage oil, avocado, betacarotene, hops extract and wheatgerm.

Testers' comments included: 'My neck, which tends to be crepey, is smooth and soft – a significant difference' • 'I'm raving about this: does more than it says on the jar' • 'cleavage in party frock wasn't as crepey' • 'neck looked less liked plucked chicken skin – with lovely sheen'.

we're not surprised that this performed well: a regenerative cream packed with antioxidants (which he swears by), including vitamins A, C and E, pomegranate and raspberry, plus ferulic acid to help fight UV damage.

Testers say: 'Top marks for this thick, rich night cream, which mostly absorbs, leaving just enough extra moisture on the

skin; skin felt smooth and really soft – closer to my own age, for a change' • 'fab texture; face feels softer than it has for a long time' • 'skin looks more dewy and feels softer and moister, so younger looking; eliminated flakiness and roughness' • 'skin looked brighter and more even' • 'fine lines finer; helped under eye; lovely'.

tried & tested
relaxing bath treats

A warm, relaxing bath is definitely cheaper than therapy – but better still when it's infused with something akin to knockout drops. Very good scores from the top contenders, in particular, which outperformed a lot of much, much more expensive bath treats.

Tisserand Lavender De-Stress Bath Soak

8.75/10 This foaming bath gel wowed our testers. But we take Tisserand to task slightly on this product, because although the word 'organic' is splashed all over the label, in reality, only the essential oils and a plant extract or two are organic, and they're blended with ammonium lauryl sulfate (which many believe is as irritating as its sister ingredient, sodium lauryl sulfate), plus cocamide DEA, neither of which we really want to see in a 'natural' product. But as we've said, our testers found that it does have tranquillity-inducing powers.

Testers say: 'Lovely, relaxing lavender smell, and with two children under two I need as much de-stressing as possible: left my very dry skin lovely and soft' • 'led to a really good night's sleep' • 'this made me feel warm and snuggly' • 'gorgeous fragrance – and I'm not a huge lavender fan; really subtle; I certainly felt more relaxed and would buy it for me, and for all my stressed-out girlfriends' • 'this product had to work hard, getting me through Christmas, flu, and husband undergoing serious op: it definitely calmed me and was very comforting: the bonus was it left my hair feeling really great'.

Organic Blue Relaxing Bath & Massage Oil ✿ ✿ ✿

8.25/10 Hats off to this Soil Association-certified organic product, which appears in our book *The Green Beauty Bible* and is your top choice if you want a truly all-natural soak (that's why we have given it the maximum quota of daisies – see page 7). It is very reasonably priced and contains oils of lavender, geranium, Roman camomile and grapefruit in a moisturising base of sunflower, jojoba and coconut oils – and can double as a massage blend.

Testers say: 'Loved it; skin felt so soft and didn't need a moisturiser

tip

You can easily make your own inexpensive relaxing bath blend: for de-stressing, put five drops of lavender, five of camomile and two of clary sage essential oils in a teaspoon, then top up with sweet almond or sunflower oil (or cream or honey); disperse in a full bath. If you have only one essential oil, make it lavender, for instant 'chill'.

for two days' • 'totally relaxed and calm after using it – wonderful sleep' • 'left me relaxed and clear headed, with soft skin' • 'fantastic value from this all-natural product, which really does the business for all-round relaxing and pampering'.

The Body Shop Divine Calm Serenity Milk Bath Powder

7.88/10 Unlike the other award winners in this category, Body Shop's comes in powder format. In running water scoops transform instantly into a milk (from soya), infused with Community Traded pure French lavender and camomile oils, which help provide a livelihood for small-scale family farmers.

Testers say: 'Wonderful: I have a very stressful job but as soon as I opened the tub, I started to relax; then I slept like a baby – and I don't often' • 'this was simple, understated and pampering' • 'I really like this: the smell is lovely, and I found it quite calming' • 'strongly scented in the tub, but nice and soothing in the water; it didn't leave a residue'.

Sanctuary Mela Amber & Tamarind Bath Nectar

7.67/10 This capsule collection from the Sanctuary spa range is inspired by India (*mela* means harmony), with exotic ingredients – and exotic packaging (though the glass bottle was deemed unsuitable by some testers). Infused with a sweet amber fragrance, this combines purifying lotus, soothing magnolia and tamarind, claimed to have 'nourishing and remineralising' properties.

Testers say: 'Wonderful extravagant aroma; made me feel lovely and relaxed as soon as I ran the bath; I would buy again, but hide from everyone!' • 'creamy smell; skin felt nourished and clean, and bath had cleaned itself!' • 'a must for any stressed mum;

divine fragrance – I could have been in a spa in Hawaii' • 'helped me sleep more soundly; skin felt soft and supple; you feel pampered' • 'poured like runny honey; lots of soft creamy bubbles, lovely smell and made me feel all relaxed and comfy; surprisingly moisturising, too' • 'would make a luxurious gift'.

Weleda Lavender Relaxing Bath Milk ❈ ❈

6.81/10 This smells powerfully of lavender, ideal (so Weleda say) 'for mental exhaustion, over-stimulation and restlessness'. They recommend enjoying its fragrant, harmonising properties at night, to promote restful sleep.

Testers say: 'Ten out of ten: I was very tired and haggard before; afterwards I felt soothed, caressed, pampered, wonderful! I had much improved, more restful sleep, with no disturbing dreams' • 'did the whole monty with this – candle, a glass of champagne – and it was a very nice, relaxing experience. It improved my sleep' • 'I like this treat as it doesn't leave the bath oily; I really like the fragrance and my weary body and mind were relaxed, uplifted and ready for sleep after using' • 'I love lavender and this felt luxurious; I slept all night after, and would buy'.

tried & tested
reviving bath treats

We'll be honest: when it comes to rev-you-up bath and shower choices, the products here (with the exception of Champneys) tailed behind pricier products. They deliver a pleasant enough experience (according to our testers), but if it's a cappuccino-esque, sense-awakening jolt you're after of a morning, stick to – well, cappuccino…

Champneys Water Mint Invigorating Shower Gel

 By far the highest scorer in this category, this is actually a moisturising body wash, with a double minty whammy of peppermint and spearmint essential oils plus uplifting orange. While not cheap-cheap, it's the most affordable of those that delivered on their boosting promises.

Testers say: 'Before shower – tired and sluggish. After shower – uplifted, refreshed and zingy!' • 'my headache went and I felt much brighter and happier!' • 'my skin felt clean, fresh, smooth and wonderfully silky afterwards' • 'I felt instantly invigorated' • 'I'm finding this slowly addictive'.

Weleda Pine Reviving Bath Milk ❋ ❋

Well done, Weleda, for such high marks in this book. A brand that's been around for over 80 years, it remains true to its biodynamic roots (ie. 'organics plus', with ingredients grown according to lunar cycles). Their bath milks were formulated 70 years ago by doctors at Weleda's health clinics. This features fir and pine (both from Siberia), and they recommend this invigorating, mountain-fresh milk after a tiring or stressful day, but also to warm you up after a cold, damp day.

Testers say: 'So pleasant: a very natural pine smell that left me relaxed and also energised; skin felt soft, too' • 'I love this natural wonder, which has rid me of prejudice against synthetic pine baths: I felt tired, uninspired and irritable and emerged refreshed, soothed and inspired, with energy' • 'great for releasing you from petty stresses and strains before a night out' • 'looks great on the shelf' • 'fab pure

we love

ingredients; skin felt soft and moisturised and very dry skin on legs not as scaly as usual' • 'not the "toilet cleaner" fragrance associated with pine; lifted my spirits and I felt re-energised'.

> If in need of a quick whoosh, we both opt for the peppermint oil trick (see 'Tip', *below*), or choose Good Works Good Morning Shower Oil, fresh-scented with rose geranium, sweet orange and ylang ylang, cunningly designed to massage into your body while you shower. You can use it in the bath, too. (Good Works is the budget cousin to This Works, and fabulous value, considering the quality of the oils and expert formulations.)

 Sainsbury's Active Naturals Lemon Verbena & Thyme Bath Milk

 A foaming bath (in a generously sized bottle, for the price), which really does have the ultra-refreshing scent of lemon verbena, in a starring role – with thyme there in the chorus. Although Sainsbury's call this range Active Naturals, there's very little that's natural in the range except the 'actives' – but the products do perform, and offer truly terrific value.

Testers say: 'The divine smell fills the bathroom and instantly calms me; I would buy it again' • 'skin felt much softer' • 'lovely, fresh, natural citrussy fragrance; instant uplifting effect. Mood lightens as soon as you step into the foam. A good size 400ml bottle, so lots of baths and quite good bubbles' • 'worked perfectly well as a shower gel; fragrance left bathroom smelling fresh and woke me up thoroughly; felt clean and fresh for a fair few hours' • 'I felt recharged but calm, and happier; one of the nicest products I have used – the packaging was appealing, too'.

Organic Surge say that the lemon, rosemary, bergamot and lime (generally thought to be sense-awakening) 'relax and calm the mind' (though, arguably, that could be reviving, couldn't it?). Anyway, we'll abide by the Beauty Bible jury's verdict…

Testers say: 'Before the bath I was tired after a bad night's sleep and long day at work; afterwards I felt relaxed and calmer and slightly energised' • 'the fragrance was lovely, uplifting and fresh smelling, and lasted the whole bath. My skin had a soft sheen, and I felt very fresh' • 'bathwater felt silky and smooth, which did create a luxurious feel' • 'left no residue or greasy feel in the bath' • 'uplifting aroma' • 'oceany, piney and refreshing: the bubbles improved my mood' • 'the bubbles were longlasting but I had to use a lot to get enough' • 'smelt natural and lemony'.

 tip

One of the fastest pick-me-ups we know is to swish ten drops of peppermint essential oil (we like Neal's Yard Remedies) in a cool-to-warm (not hot) bath. A fab way to cool down on a hot day, too.

 Organic Surge Fresh Ocean Bath Soak ✽

With a name like this, we naturally assumed it was uplifting, and sent out questionnaires accordingly. But

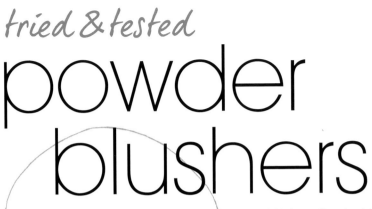

powder blushers

We've divvied blushers up into the powder version, here, and cream/gel blushers (better for more mature skins), overleaf. The powder blushers, in particular, notched up very good marks from our testers: interestingly, the top three entries are 'mineral' blushers, reflecting the shift towards all things mineral in make-up.

Prestige Skin Loving Minerals Fresh Glow Baked Minerals Blush

 Despite going to different panels of testers, the two shades of this blusher earned virtually identical scores – but Terra Rosa, a good-for-everyone soft pink, just won. Nice Perspex packaging for the price, revealing the soft-baked powder within.

Testers say: 'Lovely, slightly shimmery, peachy, goldy, pink that gave a light dusting; very natural looking' • 'went on very easily with large brush; skin looked naturally glowing' • 'better than my usual, more expensive, product; gave a smooth finish that lasted several hours' • 'Wow! What a finish! I needed quite a lot but it gave the most lovely natural glow to my skin; people kept asking if I'd been on holiday'.

  e.l.f. Mineral Blush
❋ ❋

e.l.f. is short for 'Eyes, Lips, Face' and they appear several times in this book. We can't recommend too highly that you check the range out: the pocket-money, under-a-fiver prices have to be seen to be believed. Here, a winning loose-powder 100 per cent mineral-based blusher (no parabens, no chemical dyes), trialled by our testers in Bliss – a soft-flushed pink. Not so much a steal as a SuperSteal.

Testers say: 'Easy to apply; you tip a little into the lid and swirl a blush brush into it, tap off excess and it goes on smoothly; easy to layer' • 'barely-there look, natural and pretty; compares brilliantly with my more expensive blush;

tip

The little brushes that sometimes come with blushers are almost worse than useless. Make-up pros say their thumbs are the best applicators, but we say: use a dedicated blush brush – dip it in and knock off the excess, then stroke it up your cheeks, winging it towards the temples.

exceptional quality for the price' • 'very longlasting; the first mineral make-up I've tried – and I'm impressed' • 'ideal starter blush for a teenager'.

Bourjois Little Round Pot Blush

 Wannabe-blushing beauties have turned to Bourjois since 1863. Today, this little flip-top pot of blusher – trialled in Rose Jaspe – has earned its rightful place in the Beauty Hall of Fame. Jo is totally devoted to it – she loves the pretty, sweet scent.

Testers say: 'Great texture; not too powdery, and just leaves

a gentle glow on the cheeks' • 'impressed with how good this looked: a natural glow and almost dewy look' • 'subtle rose scent, lovely finish – sheer, with a very fine sheen – a brilliant product that leaves the perfect amount of glow and colour on the cheeks. Love it!'

Revlon Matte Powder Blush

 Some of us like our blushers to have a little shimmer and glow, but this is one for shine-o-phobes. Revlon tell us that the specially coated pigments offer a soft matt look (in four shades, of which our testers had Rose Rapture) – and what we especially liked was the ingenious pop-out mirror. In general, we like a professional, fluffy brush for blusher application, but the one that comes with this isn't bad at all.

Testers say: 'Discreet shade, which you build up to the intensity required; smooth and velvety on the skin; looked very natural and glowing, with "eggshell" finish; excellent-quality brush' • 'I normally have problems with blusher, but this blended in very easily and looked natural and seamless' • 'went on beautifully and looked naturally glowing; very subtle and reasonably long lasting'.

tried & tested
cream blushers

The inexpensive cream blushers we trialled didn't have the same 'wow' factor for our testers as the powder versions. The three listed here were the best of a mixed bag: there were some truly execrable scores for other cheap cream blushers that our testers assessed. (So if you don't heed our slim list of recommendations, don't say you weren't warned.) Most cream (and gel) blushers give a light finish and are best on a bareish face, over moisturiser; they aren't designed to be rubbed over heavy foundation or concealer. Stroke them on with a foundation brush, or, as most of us do, with a finger – though some make-up artists prefer a thumb!

Max Factor Miracle Touch Creamy Blush

7/10 Don't be deceived: these Max Factor blushers may look Widow Twanky-ishly scary in the pot, but on contact with skin transform prettily from a solid colour to a sheer blush cream. They deliver a soft dewy sheen, rather than a matt finish, with a smoothness that owes a lot to castor oil – which tops the ingredient list. Max Factor suggest using it with their 'matching' Miracle Touch Foundation, but it should blend seamlessly over any liquid or cream base. Their prescribed shade was 07 Soft Candy.

Testers say: 'Love this! Went on very smoothly with my finger, and blended really well. People keep saying how healthy and glowing I look' • 'applied smoothly without dragging, and gave a smooth, sheer finish, which you can see skin through' • 'the colour looked prettiest as it started to fade: a nudge to blend it in more!' • 'absolutely love this: feels a bit sticky at first but soon disappears to give a sheer, smooth finish' • 'am constantly getting compliments about how well I look' • 'looked shockingly bright, even for my dark skin, but is much lighter on skin, and very easy to blend into a dewy, healthy, natural colour'.

we love

For an instant 'pop' of colour, instead of cream blusher we reach for our lippies, add two 'dolly' dots to cheekbones roughly in line with the outer corner of the eye, and blend well. (As always, applying a teensy bit at a time and then blending is the key to everything, make-up-wise.)

Maybelline Dream Mousse Blush

6.2/10 This has a lovely, light-as-air whipped texture, and Fiona Jolly, Maybelline's 'celebrity make-up artist', recommends: 'For perfect application, smile softly to determine the apples of your cheeks, apply the colour to this area and blend softly upwards and outwards along the cheekbone, using the tips of your fingers.' The shade tested was Mauve (really more of a soft rose, with a slight shimmer).

Testers say: 'Gave me the perfect rosy flushed glow that makes me look healthy, happy and bright' • 'easy to dip finger into whipped-cream texture – great for someone who wears little or no foundation' • 'the soft, fluffy, mousse-like texture dries to a light, powdery finish' • 'Maybelline don't test on animals – a plus for me' • 'velvety texture went on like a dream;

better than my usual, more expensive brand' • 'liked the iridescent particles, which lifted my face'.

Tecnic Whipped Blusher Mousse

6/10 Another 'whipped' option, light as air and creamy, super-blendable, from a brand just making it onto the beauty radar with fashion-forward shades, good textures and pretty amazing prices – beauty steals, every one. (As with all products in

tip

Colourwise, a good clear rosy pink or peachy blush suits most skins, with a dirty rose for 'nude skin' days, advises make-up artist Barbara Daly. (Also see page 86, for more blush advice.)

this book, you can track them down in our DIRECTORY at the back of this book, or via www.beautybible.com). There are only four shades – from deep plum to peaches-and-cream – but our testers were transformed into blushing beauties by Candy Pink. (This isn't as scary and doll like as it sounds.) It rather divided testers into 'love's and 'can't-see-the-point's'.

Testers say: 'A dream to apply – so soft and velvety – with fingers or my own brush; I came back to it day after day in preference to my own blusher because it was a soft, natural, glowing colour: two friends commented on how good my skin looked' • 'without foundation, it goes on easily and blends in seamlessly; looks glowing, due to the tiny sparkly bits; over base, goes on easily but not as glowing' • 'good compromise between cream and powder blusher' • 'you only need a very sparse amount'.

tried & tested
body butters

Mmmmm. Slurp, slurp. That's the sound of parched skin drinking in the goodness of a body butter. Ker-ching, ker-ching! That's the sound of the money you'll save with these sensational 'beauty steal' body butters: all ultra-affordable, ultra-rich, ultra-gorgeous. (And ultra-high-scoring, so we've given you four pages, with our testers' rave reviews.)

One little word of warning: according to our testers' reports, many of these products are quite highly fragranced. And the aroma can linger on – and on – and on… So do make sure you like the scent, or choose a product that is relatively unfragranced.

Yes To Carrots Deliciously Rich Body Butter ✿

9.28/10 We tested this for our book *The Green Beauty Bible*, but as it's jolly reasonably priced, it earns top place in this category, too. The rather daftly named US budget brand was a real hit with our panellists, with an exceptional score for this shea-butter-rich treatment for ultra-dry skin, which also features antioxidant ingredients derived from (yes) organic carrot juice, sweet potato, melon and pumpkin, as well as jojoba and avocado oil.

Testers say: 'Love the fresh, natural smell (not carroty!) and soft easy-to-apply texture, almost like lovely thick yogurt; skin is instantly smooth, soft and feels quenched. Love this product, and the price is incredible!'•'I would give it more than ten if I could! Was absorbed quicker than Roadrunner; pure yum, bliss to use – smelt of a cross between your mother's make-up bag when you were little and Play-Doh'•'skin looked fresh and happy'•' a joy to use, smelt heavenly, and never misbehaved'.

Boots Extracts Cocoa Butter Body Butter

 8.55/10 Very rich and creamy, and very cocoa-y. (Distinct chocolate overtones, upon massaging into skin.) Some butters in this category are light and moisture packed, and in some, the oils are more tangible – here, shea butter, sweet almond oil and cocoa butter. Boots use organic, sustainably sourced and Community Traded cocoa butter for this. Testers were divided over the aroma: most loved it; two couldn't stand it.

Testers say: 'Thick but easy to smooth in; absolutely gorgeous smell. Gave beautifully soft, silky, fragranced skin: after a week skin was softer for longer; has an expensive feel'•'big improvement in skin condition: I now have a

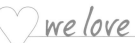

we love

Jo is now on her third pot of a fabulous and affordable product from the Dr Organic range (at Holland & Barrett): Aloe Vera Body Butter, which is light but super-hydrating and smells refreshingly citrussy. It's also very cooling on the skin (that'll be the aloe).

pot in my classroom as well as at home and all the staff use it' • 'lovely chocolatey smell! Like the wide tub; rubs in to give a slight sheen' • 'a good skin drink: went on easily, lasted the day, and skin still felt moisturised at the end' • 'ten out of ten: smells luxurious; after four days, skin felt smoother, softer and more hydrated; rough areas took a bit longer' • 'I love, love, love this product: I was going to buy a more expensive one, but this gives the same results at a fraction of the price'.

 Treacle Moon My Coconut Island Body Butter

 The first impression you get on unscrewing the lid is – well, a Bounty bar. But actually, it's not sickly: a luscious, tropically scented product with a texture that's almost jelly-like before you smooth it in to deliver a nurturing hit of shea butter. (Treacle Moon have to put a 'Please don't eat this product' on their packaging, because it all smells so edible!)

Testers say: 'Really lovely, creamy, soft product to smooth in; when it did absorb, in a couple of minutes, it felt as though it was hydrating and plumping up my

skin' • 'divine toffee-ish smell; skin was instantly plumper, shinier and felt more nourished; after a couple of days it was in fantastic condition – legs softer, smoother and had a lovely sheen' • 'A lovely product and reasonably priced' • 'I absolutely love this: itchy little bumps related to dry skin have gone – skin fantastic: I look forward to putting this on' • 'people keep asking me what it is that smells so nice'.

The Sanctuary Spa Essentials Body Butter

 Cocoa butter and creamy shea butter are the signatures of many of this category's winners, including this new entry – here, blended with sweet almond oil, macadamia oil and protective vitamin E for a decadently rich, skin-boosting treat.

Testers say: 'A most delightful body butter, with delicious smell; instantly softened and smoothed my skin and this lasted right

through the day; with constant application skin felt very supple and soft' • 'texture like whipped double cream, absorbed very quickly with no residue or stickiness; lovely fragrance' • 'after using for a week, skin feels much softer and less dry; smells great, is good value and does what it should!' • 'would make a good, inexpensive gift' • 'really smooth to apply, unlike most body butters; skin felt lovely and calm and soft – would happily use this every day'.

 Superdrug Coconut & Shea Butter Body Butter

 We have a sneaking suspicion that many of the winning products in this category are manufactured by the same contract packager: this comes in identical packaging to the Treacle Moon product, has a similar coconutty smell, feels much the same on the skin, with coconut and shea butter for instant and delicious skin nourishment (but in this case, also with *Paraffinum liquidum* – or mineral oil – at the top of the ingredient list, which one tester thought was likely to have been the cause of pore clogging).

Testers say: 'Ten out of ten: deliciously thick but easy to smooth in; not greasy or slippy; amazing smell and very silky texture; luxurious and great value for money' • 'best feature is the scent: makes me want to eat it' • 'skin stayed soft between daily uses, and can even last 48 hours' • 'reasonably priced, good, everyday product' • 'went on like silk; lush, addictive coconut smell; really works! I saw instant results on my careworn skin' • 'the best new product I have tried for years' • 'looked so thick I assumed it would "soap" on the skin, but smoothed in very easily; my skin was softer and smoother after a week, and usual dryness has disappeared'.

 Sainsbury's Active Naturals Mango & Nectarine Body Butter

 Yet another rich-textured butter at a SuperSteal price, this time subtly fragranced with apricots. The Active Naturals

range is one of Sainsbury's most enduringly successful beauty lines: simple, no-nonsense products with some very nice smells indeed.

Testers say: 'Lovely, buttery rich and conditioning; absorbed quickly; divine smell; instant hydrated skin with a lovely glow; impressive, excellent value for money – my daughter loved it, too' • 'surprisingly easy to apply, compared to other body butters; ten out of ten for lasting fragrance; looked like a freshly made mango fool – very appealing! Performs as well as a more expensive product' • 'skin felt smooth and soft and effects lasted a good few hours'.

 Beautifully Delicious Butterlicious Coconut & Shea Body Butter

 Well, well, well: looks like the product from Superdrug and Treacle Moon, smells like those skin treats, has a similar texture – and, as with Treacle Moon, there's a 'Do not eat!' warning on the packaging. And – guess what? – it went down almost as well with our testers. The bottom line? A great product is a great product, whichever brand it's under.

Testers say: 'This product is so creamy and wonderful; absorbed very quickly, in seconds. Very luxurious texture; you get wonderfully smooth skin on application, which lasted on hands, despite washing up' • 'since using this scrumptious cream on my feet, I shall be showing them off in sandals this summer' • 'I'd definitely buy this, and have recommended it to friends' • 'skin noticeably smoother, with a nice sheen; there is something luxurious about a big pot of creamy butter and I really enjoyed the ritual of putting it on' • 'ten out of ten: smells gorgeous; when I opened the jar at work colleagues all demanded to try it' • 'I enjoyed using this and my normally dry skin is soft and smooth after a week, with no tightness or flakiness'.

Tisserand Nourishing Body Butter ❀

This lavender, sweet orange and bergamot butter also wowed our 'greener' testers. It's a lovely product, but we do wish Tisserand wouldn't keep banging on about their products being organic on the packaging when basically it's just the oils and extracts rather than the bulk ingredients – in this case, shea butter, cocoa butter, *tip* **We never throw an avocado skin away without turning it inside out and smoothing the last traces of pulp over forearms and the backs of hands. Yes, it's a bit green to start with, but as you smooth it in, that tinge disappears, leaving skin fabulously nourished – as a gift-with-purchase!**

sweet almond, olive and sunflower oils – which are certified sustainable. Several testers thought it meant the whole product was organic, which it's not.

Testers say: 'Smooths in very quickly, straight from the pot; doesn't feel greasy or oily; left skin scented and moisturised, softer and more cared for, with a nice healthy glow' • 'looked quite high end; skin smelt nice and was instantly glowing' • 'very skin friendly, and although my skin is sensitive, it was fine after shaving my legs' • 'a good product, and the price suits my purse strings: made sure my skin was flake-free during some of the most windswept and cold months' of the year • 'used it after showering daily and skin lost that grey winter pallor: within a week I found that I needed to use less and skin wasn't so obviously thirsty'.

Organic Surge Fresh Ocean Body Butter ✿

 Frankly, what makes you fall in love with a product is usually the smell – and this is one for anyone who loves a fresh, more 'ozonic' scent, derived from aromatic essential oils. Almost a mousse-like texture to this luscious body treat, which cocoons skin with avocado, rosehip, shea butter and cocoa butter; they suggest it's ideal for use on skin that's tender after shaving or waxing.

Testers say: 'Skin feels plumper, soft and silky – my husband and children commented on that!' • 'one of the better moisturisers, which gives instant hydration but doesn't take any time to dry; leaves no oily residue and is effective' • 'very pleasant, light moussey consistency – like whipped cream; skin feels moisturised immediately' • 'ten out of ten! Fantastic smell,

lemony rosemary – love it: this was absorbed very quickly, but has longlasting effects; I have bought more and will continue to do so'.

Champneys Moisture Miracle Skin Comforting Body Butter

 One of the richest options in this category, with an ultra-creamy texture: another galumphing great tub offering up a blend of shea, olive, mango and cocoa butters, plus added lingonberry oil, rich in Omega-3 fatty acids. (The geranium, orange and cedarwood fragrance is more sophisticated and 'grown up' than some in this category, which have more 'teen appeal'.)

Testers say: 'Ten out of ten: absorbed immediately; sweet, natural (ie, not chemical) scent. Very pleasant to use: soft enough to scoop easily with fingers, and moisturises very well all over, including problem areas – superb!' • 'as a nurse I'm on my knees a lot (don't ask!) and they get very dry and flakey; I usually put Vaseline on, but with this cream I didn't have to do that' • 'absorbs more quickly than most body butters and leaves skin feeling soft without stickyness'.

tried & tested
body lotions

As with body butters, our testers were super-keen on a lot of entries in this category – so the results stretch over four pages. We trialled a list of products as long as your arm (and leg) – more than 100 in all – and these fabulously high-scoring winners did better than many, many more expensive options. (We tend to use butters for hands, elbows, feet, knees, with lotions for the rest of the body – on areas of skin that aren't so thick-skinned and thirsty.)

Yes to Carrots C is Smooth Body Moisturizing Lotion ❀

8.7/10 Not quite as stupendously high scoring as its 'sister' body butter (see page 24), but still a worthy winner of this category. The 'signature' ingredients of this rich lotion are organic carrot juice, pumpkin, sweet potato and melon. (To our noses, the fragrance is baby powderish, by the way – and rather comforting, for that.) As a natural product, it also appears in our 'green' tome.

Testers say: 'Ten out of ten, for light creamy texture; immediately absorbed; good packaging; skin immediately moisturised and comfy; with regular use skin felt more healthy and supple' • 'slightly disappointed that it doesn't smell of carrots! But like the light, fresh fragrance and silky lotion; excellent packaging, gave softer skin and areas of dryness improved; I am very impressed' • 'really enjoyed using this; quickly absorbed and very effective'.

Jergens Naturals Age Defying
Body Moisturiser ❈

 There are high levels of natural ingredients in this new-to-the-UK collection of four products from one of the States' bestselling bodycare brands (all performed well in our trials). With green tea extract, this promises 'younger-looking skin in two weeks'. The fresh fragrance is down to mint and sage.

Testers say: 'Very easy to swoosh on; nice fresh, green smell; made my skin radiantly soft and moisturised' • 'great affordable effective product; absorbed very quickly; excellent for everyday use' • 'lovely silky lotion; skin was smooth looking and felt more comfortable instantaneously! Wow!' • 'I needed a few days to fall in love, but, as with a good man, it was worth being patient for – and I am no longer a dried-up old prune, wayhey!' • 'like the fact that it has pictures on the label that show it is cruelty free, low carbon, etc – and I am very impressed with softness'.

Good Works Good Looking Body Lotion ❈

A very sophisticated blend of high-quality essential oils – including palmarosa, geranium and patchouli – makes this heaven for the senses, while a pump-action bottle delivers a nourishing blend based on olive and sunflower oils. We applaud the fact that Good Works – set up by our ex-*Vogue* beauty director friend Kathy Phillips – keenly supports the Kids Company charity with proceeds raised by the range. Feels good, smells good, does good.

Testers say: 'Very nice, creamy, expensive-feeling product which gave me smoother, softer skin instantly; feels very good on your skin – I would recommend it' • 'this was heaven for me; smells divine and sank in instantly, so skin felt hydrated immediately; everything about it was great – an ideal product' • 'I felt so feminine: the smell of this is very sensual and my skin was almost velvety' • 'very good body lotion with lovely fresh smell; I enjoyed using this'.

Marks & Spencer Formula Super Hydrating Body Cream Oil

 Cream-oils are just that: they go on like a cream, sink in like an oil, leaving skin supple and nourished with a soft sheen. Humectant glycerine gives this its moisture power, with olive and sunflower oils in the formulation (although somewhat behind the petrolatum and mineral oil on the ingredients list, once we'd got out the magnifying glass to inspect it).

Testers say: 'This is my beauty find: an unassuming product that has beaten all rivals I have used hands down, does what it says and has brought pleasure to what's usually a chore!' • 'I feel I've

---

♡ *we love*

We both adore the Good Looking Body Lotion from Good Works (*above*) and agree this is as fabulous a blend of essentials oils as you'll find in any product, at any price. For us, it's always down to fragrance, as much as texture – though we like the richness of this, too.

traded in my tired skin for something more youthful, soft, radiant and comfortable'•'an absolute delight to put on; gorgeous smell, reminiscent of childhood; skin felt lovely all over'•'skin instantly moisturised, with a nice sheen'.

 ### Garnier Skin Naturals Hydralock Moisturising Milk

 A gargantuan bottle of super-hydrating milk, which Garnier promise delivers 'non-stop hydration 24 hours' (and Jo thinks it lives up to that, having got through a bottle soothing stubbornly dry winter shins). They also claim it will 'visibly transform skin in one week', partly thanks to five per cent hydro-urea – a high level of this well-known moisturising ingredient.

Testers say: 'This worked instantly for me; parched skin was nourished and almost dewy; by day three, even the driest areas looked well nourished and satiny; they claim skin is visibly transformed in eight days – this was true, and in a much shorter time scale'•'an absolute winner'•'surprised I could use this on my sensitive skin; also smoothed the *keratosis pilaris* [rough bumps, aka chicken skin] on my upper arms – a plus!'•'really liked the fresh, light smell, like freshly washed clothes'.

 ### Aveeno Skin Relief Body Lotion

 Aveeno have built a reputation on soothing and quenching dry skin, with a range that incorporates calming ingredients like colloidal oatmeal, clinically proven to moisturise for 24 hours, together with natural emollients and moisturisers such as shea butter, plus vitamins A and E. There are many skin soothers in the Aveeno range, including this – which does have a whiff-of-porridge scent to it (in a nice way), but to our nostrils seems otherwise unfragranced.

Testers say: 'An absolute winner, which I will definitely buy again – great feel, easily absorbed and genuinely works; nondescript fragrance; fairly natural'•'much improved dry skin areas immediately; after a few days, generally much softer and smoother, and did keep skin hydrated all day'•'absorbed into skin like a dream; really nice creamy texture; would definitely buy this, I loved it so much and it's a great price: I also used it on my little boy's dry skin patches and it really improved his skin too'.

Tisserand Vitamin Rich Body Lotion

 Mango butter delivers the moisture power in this, which has a powerful antioxidant blend of green tea, vitamins C and E, plus conditioning pro-vitamin B5. A 'euphoric citrus aroma' is how Tisserand describe the fragrance, which has plenty of jasmine, sweet orange and orange leaf oil.

Testers say: 'Lovely natural smell of oranges; gave smooth, soft skin immediately'•'very easy to use: no sooner applied than it sinks in; very rich looking and feeling – beautiful aroma; skin moisturised and softened: I looked forward to using this'•'left skin lightly moisturised and smell was uplifting'•'skin looked more healthy and hydrated, the longer I used it – really liked this product, and I would use it regularly'•'I would buy this as a gift'.

Champneys Vitamiracle Ultra Smooth Body Lotion

Somehow, this pulls off the trick of being lightweight but very nourishing. Key ingredients are vitamins A, C and E, smoothing papaya extract, plus moisturising meadowfoam seed oil. It's from the Champneys range, formulated in tandem with their spa team, which is used in their treatments – but it is also available at Sainsbury's, where the range has become a worthy bestseller.

Testers say: 'Ten out of ten: quite rich, but absorbed very quickly; no overt smell, which is good. Immediate softness, dreaded elbow redness reduced, lumpy bits on arms better; fish-scale on shins gone after a few days and skin stays smoother longer' • 'I really like this; very easy to smooth in; not greasy– you can dress pretty much immediately; light, warm fragrance; left skin noticeably softer, smoother, silky to touch; general moisture levels improved after a week' • 'really good moisturiser to mix with fake tan' • 'I loved this and will give up my usual cream; the smell comforted me; the lotion soaked in and left skin soft and silky: I am buying more!'

  Jergens Naturals Ultra Hydrating Body Moisturiser ❀

7.66 / 10 Another Jergens winner: slightly richer than the 'age-defying' option which came higher up our charts, and powered here by jojoba oil – a renowned nourisher. This has a very subtle 'ozonic' scent. Again,

tip

'In winter, give hands and arms a deep treat by applying a heavy moisturiser from fingertips to your elbow, then wrapping them in clingfilm. After 20 minutes, discard the clingfilm and rub in the excess cream.' Ji Baek, Rescue Beauty Lounge

this sinks in fast, but delivers enduring moisturisation.

Testers say: 'I would definitely buy this: very easy to smooth in; smells gently fragrant; my skin felt instantly smooth and hydrated; after a few days my elbows are smoother, and generally skin feels moisturised, even when I haven't yet applied the lotion' • 'a great eight out of ten for this light, silky lotion from an eczema and psoriasis sufferer! Left skin dewy and moist on first application; after a few days my skin was generally softer and more supple, more toned as dry blotchy areas reduced and skin was better long term' • 'really helped with scaly skin on legs after shaving'.

Dove ProAge Body Cream Oil

7.6 / 10 Another cream-oil: formulated for especially dry skin (and from the range targeted at women over 45), this has a high glycerine content, together with skin-conditioning olive oil (and *Paraffinum liquidum*, aka mineral oil, which some testers would have preferred not to have been included), but is non-greasy.

Testers say: 'The immediate effect of this was good, and after a few days, there was a definite improvement in skin condition; smelt fine, a bit like baby powder; I really liked it' • 'wasn't sticky or greasy; skin feels softer and I have fewer ingrowing hairs after depilating' • 'moisturises really well; having just had surgery, I was pleasantly surprised to see an improvement in the scar on my abdomen: an inexpensive but very effective body cream for all ages, though sadly my teenage daughters wouldn't use it because of the name' • 'a little goes a long way, and after applying this at night, my skin had a lovely softness in the morning' • 'skin smooth and velvety to touch; I will buy and use this daily'.

tried & tested
body oils

Frankly, if you want a really cheap body oil you can just slap on something you'd use for cooking (sunflower and olive oil are both terrific nourishers). Looking for something with a higher pleasure quotient? Our testers appreciatively slurped up lots of the body oil 'steals' we sent out…

The Body Shop Spa Wisdom Monoi Miracle Oil ❀

 This rich blend nudges in under the tenner mark, with its blissful tropical fragrance – from monoi (Tahitian gardenia flowers); it also made it into *The Green Beauty Bible* because of its plant content. It delivers skin nourishment from coconut and babassu oils (the babassu coming from The Body Shop's Community Trade Project, giving 12 rural communities of women the opportunity for regular work).
Testers say: 'Smells like heaven and was a treat to use'•'gave a dewy shimmer, wonderful scent and softness to skin'•'worked magic in patches of dry skin'• 'worked amazingly as a hair oil, left overnight'•'fab applied before big night out: made skin glowy'.

Neutrogena Natural Sesame Seed Body Oil

 This is a true beauty classic – based on real sesame oil, not mineral oil (which many inexpensive body oils are made up of). It was especially formulated for dry, sensitive skin – and an 'insider tip' for use is to slurp it on in the shower, or apply to just-damp skin.
Testers say: 'I love this! It's like fabric softener for the skin… Being able to smother myself in it straight out of the shower was an easy habit, and I just loved the velvety skin and gorgeous smell' •'my skin had a healthy glow and was immediately softer; beneficial particularly for dry areas, like knees and elbows' •'gave a nice sheen and softness; absorbed quickly – I loved the non-greasiness: a great addition to the bath, too'.

Elle Macpherson Self Calming Bath & Body Oil

 We're keen on any product that does double duty: some body oils aren't suitable for bath use because they just sit on the surface without diffusing (drip them under a running tap to overcome this, or mix with milk, cream or honey), but this can be infused immediately into hot water for a relaxing soak – and spritzed on to the body, allowing you to surrender to its subtle lavender scent.

Testers say: 'My skin had a satin sheen, so looked extra special – a wee confidence boost and psychological pick-me-up' • 'dry areas were instantly improved' • 'absorbed quite quickly, smelt strongly of lavender, which I like – main effect was feeling pampered and relaxed' • 'didn't notice major improvement in dryness but it did help me sleep!' • 'loved the funky packaging. Good for my sensitive skin; really good value for money – though I would prefer that it didn't use petrochemicals' • 'not an original scent, but deeply relaxing – so much so, I nearly didn't get out of a midday bath for a meeting'.

Weleda Lavender Relaxing Body Oil ✿✿

6.66/10 A relatively new introduction from Weleda, this product is your top choice if you're looking for a 100 per cent natural body oil (also for use as a massage and bath oil). This is based on organic sesame oil and sweet almond oil, and (like Elle's, *left*) is especially good for helping to soothe the senses before bedtime, thanks to the extracts

♡ we love

Jo's been a fan of the nourishing-but-sinks-in-fast Neutrogena Natural Sesame Seed Body Oil for years. (She unscrews the top and adds 20 drops of sweet orange essential oil and 20 drops of patchouli, to sex up the understated fragrance.) She also likes Weleda Sea Buckthorn Body Oil, in which sesame is also a star ingredient – a 'sister' product to the lavender version which scored well here. Sarah makes her own concoctions with sweet almond oil, and a few drops of essential oils, such as rose and patchouli. (Almost as cheap as olive oil… another huge favourite.)

of organic lavender incorporated in the formula.

Testers say: 'This is best used after a bath, when the skin is warm and pliant; it sank into my thirsty skin very quickly – I put on tights immediately afterwards, and the oil didn't ooze through' • 'this left my skin with a sexy sheen, according to my husband' • 'I loved the fact that this product can also be used as a massage and bath oil'.

Botanics Organic Nourishing Body Oil ✿✿

6.61/10 All-organic (but not certified – despite what looks like a proper organic 'seal' on the packaging), this rich oil has a jojoba base (so it pours s-l-o-w-l-y from the bottle, rather than whooshes out). It's delicately fragranced with a blend of rose, geranium and bergamot oils, which we – and our testers – really loved.

Testers say: 'Skin felt deeply moisturised and more supple, smoother and nourished; particularly smoothed top of arms, improved crepiness on lower legs and was great overnight on my dry feet' • 'very easy to smooth into skin and was absorbed very quickly; lovely light, fruity fragrance; skin felt supple and had a lovely sheen; effects built up over seven to ten days to give flake-less soft skin' • 'really liked this light oil, though would prefer pump dispenser to glass bottle' • 'got my husband to massage my back with this, which was a definite plus!'

tried & tested
body scrubs

Knowing that our testers are a real bunch of scrubbers (in the nicest possible way), we dispatched a couple of dozen different body-buffing 'steals' to them. Their favourites – featured here – scored quite considerably better than the rest of the products trialled: seems there are some duff scruffs out there, but these definitely aren't among them.

FCUK
Sugarscrub

If you like your products scented with (wild) strawberry, you'll love this. (And if you don't, well…) Richly textured, it features larger sugar granules for a super-buffing action, suspended in jojoba and sweet almond oils, with a generous dollop of shea butter, to leave skin hydrated.

Testers say: 'Ten out of ten for this! The nicest ever smell, a pleasure to use; the sugar particles were so gentle; sloughs away dead skin and rough areas, leaving a supple, shiny finish – perfect!' • 'great

cheap bathroom staple – don't be a skincare snob or you'll miss out' • 'my spotty arms and very dry elbows felt nicely moisturised and smoother; loved the look, too; would happily leave it on show'.

The Sanctuary Hot Sugar Body Polish

There was a national outcry when The Sanctuary discontinued this polish – so it was reintroduced! Massaged into the skin, the self-heating gel has an intriguing warming action to help stimulate the circulation. The skin-scruffing action is

down to organic sugar.

Testers say: 'A dream to use: easy to apply and to wash off – the heat element made it very soothing; left skin moisturised and smooth' • 'no dry or dull patches anywhere after using this; skin felt buffed and ready for my next batch of tan' • 'I had no ingrowing hairs after waxing' • 'the bumps that plague my arms are feeling much less raised since I've been using this'.

Garnier Bodytonic Sugar Scrub

Garnier say this is 'enriched with natural ingredients', but sugar features a l-o-n-g way down the list (after sodium lauryl sulfate and propylene glycol, to name but two, in what one tester described as a 'chem lab list'). Nevertheless, the lightly foaming formulation does leave skin super-smooth and super-soft, with whispers of the signature lemon fragrance. (We'd almost categorise this as a body wash with buffing bits.)

Testers say: 'My dull, dry skin felt coated in a moisturising protective film; much smoother and softer; very good price point' • 'skin looked a little brighter than usual' • 'I could use the squeezy bottle easily with one hand, and the fresh-smelling scrub washed off as easily as soap; my skin felt smoother and softer from the first use – better than my expensive brand' • 'I like everything about this product, and will buy it again'.

Elle Macpherson Bare Double Duty Cleanse & Scrub

 This product swooshes skin clean and exfoliates, all in one, with a skin-softening and moisturising action due to the glycerine in the formula. Elle has been quoted as saying that it's her favourite within the whole range, which has three 'sub-categories': this is from 'Bare' – the daily must-haves – while

'Self' is 'me time' and 'Glow' is for going out.

Testers say: 'Really like this and it's great value – easy-to-use gel, perfect texture – grainy but not coarse; washed off easily, leaving skin smooth and moisturised' • 'delicious smell that was really energising; surprisingly moisturising – transformed my suffering skin' • 'I like a scrub to do what it says on the tin – and this one delivers'.

Champneys Citrus Glow Hydrating Sugar Scrub

This 'ties' with Elle's scrub: its scruffing power comes from demerara and organic brown sugars plus coconut fibres, to leave skin moisturised as well as brighter. The scent's particularly lovely: alongside fresh lemony notes you'll encounter a warm cardamom spiciness. (Has played a starring role in Jo's bathroom, at various times.)

tip

Should you ever pitch up at your holiday destination and find you haven't packed a body scrub, grab a few freebie packets of salt from a food takeaway. Either combine with a body wash or any oil, or use on slightly dampened skin, working in gentle circles – especially on knees, elbows, upper arms. (For feet, you can make do with wet sand, on the beach.)

Testers say: 'Smells divine; I wanted to eat it – good texture, like wet sand, left my skin feeling soooo soft and lovely; a real treat' • 'smells lovely, feels lovely, and isn't too expensive, so I will buy again and recommend to my friends – I love it so much!' • 'smelt of Thornton's Sicilian lemon mousse chocs – lovely; skin looked pink and healthy with a nice sheen, and very moisturised; could shave legs without foam' • 'easy to get the product out of the tub and you don't need to use a lot'.

'The one piece of beauty advice I would give is exfoliate, exfoliate, exfoliate. It's the only way to keep skin soft, smooth and glowing.'

ELLE MACPHERSON

tried & tested
body washes

We almost drowned in entries for this category: body washes (which just happen to work equally well as shower gels) seem to be one of the fastest-growing areas of beauty products. (R.I.P. soap!) In general, a high-scoring category, with testers especially loving these ones.

Yes to Carrots C How to Shower Carrot Rich Shower Gel ❀

8.25/10 'Twenty-six Dead Sea minerals purify the skin to nourish and revive', promise kookily named Yes to Carrots (YTC), while sweet almond, olive and jojoba oil ensure the wash isn't at all drying. What also makes this a steal is the HUGE bottle – half a litre of the gently bubbling stuff.

Testers say: 'Skin felt nice after use, no tightness or dryness – and no scary ingredients' • 'just the right foaminess; rinsed off easily; liked the fashionable packaging' • 'loved this – even my fussy husband did; it's bright orange and smells fruity – not carroty! – made me feel happy' • 'pleasure to bathe with this and it suited my daughter's very sensitive skin; the smell and softness of the water (in a very hard water area) were fabulous – hard to beat for value'.

The Sanctuary Amla & Cardamom Shower Drench

8/10 According to Hindu tradition, 'the mother goddess nourishes mankind with the fruits of the amla tree'. This Indian fruit is certainly packed with vitamin C, and here is combined in a creamy wash with fragrant jasmine, aromatic cardamom and gotu kola herb. The Sanctuary promise it's 'as refreshing to the spirit as the tranquil gardens of an Indian palace' – and here's what our testers thought…

Testers say: 'Ten out of ten! Loved this creamy wash – and the smell! It felt luxurious and the scent was 'enveloping' – kept sniffing my arms' • 'only needed a little, and rinsed off well with no residue; although there's a long list of chemicals, it's paraben-free and not tested on animals' • 'very good flip-top packaging; left skin moisturised and fresh. I would definitely buy this'.

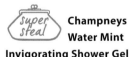 **Champneys Water Mint Invigorating Shower Gel**

7.12/10 This also features under Uplifting Bath Treats (see page 19), but it's done well as a body wash/shower gel too. Its wake-up power comes from a blend of peppermint, spearmint and orange, in a gentle, amino acid, pH-balanced cleanser.

Testers say: 'Before shower – tired and sluggish. After shower – uplifted, refreshed and zingy!' • 'the headache which had been nagging me went and I felt much brighter and happier!' • 'my skin felt clean, fresh, smooth and silky afterwards' • 'I felt instantly invigorated and knew I was going to have a great night out!' • 'I'm finding this slowly addictive'.

  Dr. Organic Bioactive Skincare 100% Organic Tea Tree Body Wash

 From Holland & Barrett's ultra-reasonably priced natural bodycare range (with high levels of organically certified ingredients), a tea tree-based product which is good for anyone suffering from breakouts and acne on body skin – thanks to tea tree's ability to unblock pores and balance excess oil, plus its anti-bacterial action.

Testers say: 'Love the fragrance: really good wash scent – antiseptic, clean and natural; foams just the right amount; a little went a long way; easy to

---

rinse off, and left a lovely tingling fresh feeling from the mint' • 'my male partner liked the very fresh awakening fragrance in the mornings' • 'almost tingled on my skin – left it feeling clean but softer and slightly smoother than usual, which was a nice surprise – I really love this'.

Purely Skincare Organic Grapefruit & Lemongrass Shower Gel ❀ ❀

A micro-point behind Dr. Organic comes a natural creation from a range specifically formulated to be free from SLS and SLES, artificial colours, parabens and petrochemicals – which the brand's founder had established made his father-in-law's rosacea worse. (Rosacea's not just a girl thing.) The zesty citrus scent is a great morning wake-up call.

Testers say: 'Foams really well and you can smell the grapefruit and lemongrass for a long time

---

after use; only needed a little and it rinsed off easily' • 'an efficient cleanser with a zesty smell' • 'liked the citrussy fragrance, which woke me up in the morning' • 'using it with the loofah or bath puff really helped it foam enough to shave my legs with; reasonably priced, very nice product' • 'I do a lot of running and used it after; I really think it helped my achey legs!'

tip

Body washes double as fantastic lingerie washes, too: squirt into a basin of warm water (no hotter), swish with your hands and you've found a much kinder way to get your bras clean. Rinse well and dry naturally.

tried & tested
bronzers

Once upon a time, you could tell an inexpensive bronzing powder: the textures were scratchy, the shades somewhat sunburned. Not any more: our testers (who trialled more than 20 in total) were generally pretty happy with the way these kiss skin with a touch of sun, delivering a seamless finish. (Other entries fared less well, please note.)

L'Oréal Glam Bronze Blush Duo

 This bronzer stormed into first place, trailing the other winners some distance behind: it's a clever two-in-one powder compact which is half bronzer, half pretty pink blusher. (Our testers tried the 301 Blondes shade; there is also an option for Brunettes.) You can use the two halves separately, or swirl them together to customise a subtly shimmering, healthy, all-over glow. There's an integral mirror and quite a generous brush in the base (though we'd always recommend bigger brushes; see page 8).

Testers say: 'Would give this more than ten, if I could! Very portable, though best applied with a big not-so-portable brush – I swirled the two colours together, which gave my pale skin a lovely glow, and left it still surprisingly dewy looking' • 'very good summer substitute!' • 'very fine and light; went on very evenly' • 'gave a glowing, shimmery effect on my face, including eyelids (the bronze) and décolletage' • 'lovely creamy powder that gave a dewy finish, and lasted as long as I needed'.

 e.l.f. Healthy Glow Bronzing Powder

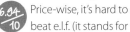 Price-wise, it's hard to beat e.l.f. (it stands for Eyes, Lips, Face), who have a winner here with this simple see-through Perspex powder compact. The formulation itself is more shimmering than some, so probably not the ideal choice if you've a tendency to shine – but the texture is sublimely silky-soft, and the shade our panellists got to try – 2401 Sun Kissed – is said to 'complement any skintone'.

Testers say: 'Fine silky powder, which blended easily and gave a lovely sunkissed look – I'm a convert!' • 'surprisingly flattering; I hated the look of it but once I managed to open it and popped it on, I really loved it' • 'discreetly sheeny finish that leaves your face healthy, glowing and sunkissed – a real treat; it looks as if I've caught some sun without getting any of the damage'

• 'colour lasted all day' • 'I wasn't impressed at first, but this grew on me; best to load brush with bronzer, flick off excess, then stroke it on'.

Rimmel Natural Bronzer

 Twist off the lid and you'll find a light, natural-looking bronzing powder – it comes in just one shade, 021 Sun Light. Although it's not enough to shield skin on a summer day or if you're spending a lot of time outside, Rimmel tell us this offers an SPF8, for some degree of temporary, light sun protection.

Testers say: 'Lovely texture – fine and silky; very easy to use; blended evenly and smoothly – didn't "sit" on the skin; gave a subtle healthy glow, slightly matt, slightly dewy – just about right' • 'this lasted from breakfast to lunch, then needed a little

touching up' • 'powder blended well when I brushed it on, and was subtle enough to build up for more "glow"; being a bronzer beginner, I had a massive fear of looking orange and ridiculous, but this turned out to be really great' • 'has changed the way I use make up: now I use this when I have been having a "tired" day – so thank you!'.

GOSH Precious Powder Pearls

 Guerlain pioneered 'bronzing pearls' a couple of decades ago with their ultra-luxe Météorites range, and the concept has now trickled down to the mass market. This GOSH product comes in just one shade (Glow) – you swirl a soft brush gently over the vari-shaded pearls, collecting just the right amount to apply to the skin, dusting on to cheekbones, forehead, chin and décolletage. One warning: keep them on your

dressing table at home, to avoid make-up bag disasters (if the lid comes off, the crushed beads get into everything).

Testers say: 'This is a real gem! I couldn't believe it was a cheap brand – silky, rich powder that blended beautifully and sat really well on my skin' • 'works equally well on bare skin or over foundation; gives a matt finish with a subtle shimmer; I'm really surprised by how much I like this product' • 'I really like the effect; this gave a soft glow on my very fair skin; at night I used it on shoulders and chest – I've even used it in daytime on bare skin, and I look healthy and not orange!' • 'I thought bronzers would look unnatural on my pale skin, but now I'm a convert'.

---

tip

To avoid patchiness, allow at least 15 minutes for moisturiser to sink in before applying bronzing powder, for a can't-tell-it-from-tanned perfect finish.

♡ *we love*

Jo fakes a summer glow with Bourjois Mineral Radiance, in a lightly sunkissed shade called Hâlé, which features micronised quartz to boost radiance (and make-up artist Jenny Jordan recommends it, too; see feature on page 86).

tried & tested
brow pencils

As a blonde, Jo knows exactly how vital brow pencil is: without it, she disappears. A few deft pencil strokes, and hey, presto! Jo's back. But whatever your skin tone, brow pencil can make for an instant groomed look (think how crucial Audrey Hepburn's brows were to her 'look').

Just as we always suspected: our testers found the 'steals' they tried rivalled the very expensive brands, with the winner coming a micro-point behind a Dior product, but at a tenth of the price. (Ssshhh! We didn't tell you that!)

Collection 2000 Eyebrow Definer

You'd never guess from the rather understated, workaday design of this basic pencil that it would prove a decisive winner. For some bizarre reason it comes in just two shades – Blonde and Black, with nothing in between those two extremes. However, Collection 2000 sent us both to try: this score is for Blonde, and Black did quite well too, with 6.75/10.

Testers say: 'Very easy to apply, especially as I am an eyebrow pencil virgin. I was surprised at how excited I am about this product; it is really great – I am surprised that my brows appear more defined and lifted' • 'it went on smoothly, no dragging, and was easy to apply precisely when used properly – though it took me a while to perfect the technique; it did look natural' • 'easy to apply precisely – stayed put for six to eight hours' • 'I am going to try to convert my Mum: she has overplucked in the past'.

Soap & Glory Arch de Triumph

Is there no end to our friend Marcia Kilgore's ingenuity? Seemingly not. This stubby pencil means business. At one end, you'll find a soft pencil in a shade that seems to suit and enhance every shade of brow. But at the other, there's a brow highlighting pencil: applied to the brow-bone, it has a real eye-opening, almost 'face-lifting' effect. You do need to buy a special big sharpener but it comes with fun stencils to guide your arching!

we love

Soap & Glory Arch de Triumph, for its clever design (and because the name puts a smile on both our faces). Jo also rates the Clinique Superfine Liner for Brows, which comes in at just under our price ceiling: it's an ultra-slim, automatic pencil with a super-fine tip so it never needs sharpening. And the Soft Blonde colour is ideal.

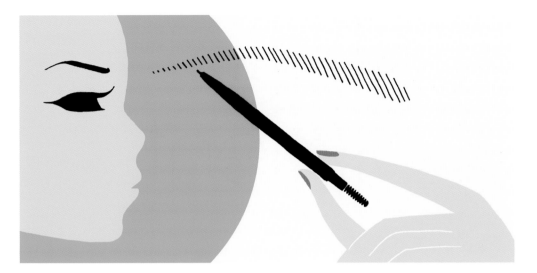

Testers say: 'Lovely to use; goes on really nicely; easy to apply a precise shape – and if you make a mistake you can rub the pencil on your skin, and remove it easily. I love it' • 'I can create an eyebrow shape like Kylie Minogue, and having plucked my eyebrows to oblivion in the 1980s, having natural full eyebrows is a joy' • 'texture very good; lasted about seven hours; the best eyebrow pencil I've tried' • 'created a very natural fuller brow effect' • 'brows looked perfect all day'.

 Rimmel Professional Eyebrow Pencil

7.14/10 Why professional? Probably because this comes with a built-in brush, for brow-grooming both before and after you make light, feathery strokes with the pencil. (That's what pros do.) It comes in a few shades; our testers had Hazel 002, the lightest.

Testers say: 'I would definitely buy this; I had been using another brand, but this is a great product and great value for money' • 'pretty easy to be precise, just using the same principle as writing; good staying power and lasted all day' • 'looked very natural; the perfect colour for me; very slim tip enabled very precise application' • ' not only is this cheaper than the brow pencils I use, but it looks more natural and stays on longer, too' • 'good for light brows – and it comes with a brush'.

No 7 Precision Brow Pencil

7.06/10 With the 'propelling pencil' type, like this one, there's no risk that you'll scratch fragile skin with a pencil worn down to its wooden stump. It has a slanted tip so it's easy to get the right angle, and comes in a whisker under our price 'ceiling'. Three shades; we trialled Brown.

Testers say: 'Quite easy to use once you got the hang of the wedge-shaped pencil; generally looked more natural than most brow pencils' • 'very easy to apply' • 'my 85-year-old mother is totally delighted with this for her sparse eyebrows – the ease of use, effectiveness and smoothness of the pencil are important' • 'easy to apply and a good natural colour; best quality I have used'.

tried & tested
cellulite treatments

This really is one of the biggest beauty woes – and so one of the biggest challenges. Can any product truly work to improve the appearance of dimples, and flabbiness of thighs and derrière? Surprisingly, the answer seems to be 'yes' – and some of the highest-scoring products we've ever trialled happen to be at rock-bottom prices.

NB: most of these products come with instructions on how to massage in for best results: we recommend following them. The tester who just wanted the product to work miracles on its own because following the instructions was 'a pain' (though she admitted they were quite straightforward) gets *nul points* **– and got** *nul* **improvement, too.**

Weleda Birch Cellulite Oil ❀❀

8.28/10 This is one of the most effective cellulite products we've ever trialled – and it's all natural. The circulation-boosting elements are derived from young organic birch leaves, rosemary and ruscus, in a base of wheatgerm and jojoba which you massage into the cellulite-affected areas – and as our testers report, it really does deliver impressive results. It's designed to be used in tandem with other cellulite busters in the Weleda range, but our testers got these results from using this product alone.

Testers say: 'Following the clear instructions for this attractive smelling oil, my skin feels much smoother and more refined; texture is better and cellulite look not gone but much improved • 'sank in quickly, improved skin texture making it softer, smoother and less bumpy' • 'good value' • 'I'm really sceptical about cellulite products but this one is worth continuing with, alongside regular exercise, etc'.

Nivea Body Goodbye Cellulite

7/10 The active ingredient in this skin-smoothing cream-gel is l-carnitine, an amino acid involved in the breakdown of fat. This butt-blitzer is a phenomenal success story, top of the anti-cellulite charts in France, Italy, Belgium, Turkey, Portugal and the Netherlands. It is priced very slightly above our usual 'ceiling' of a tenner.

Testers say: 'Easy-spread gel, quickly absorbed with a circular rub-in motion: simple instructions; skin much softer and brighter, more uniformly white, less bumpy: improved the appearance of cellulite – after a week, visible difference on back of thigh and bottom' • 'skin less dimpled, more toned, less exercise!' • 'not sticky – so am not a fluff magnet' • 'definitely recommend it – perfect' • 'thighs feel firmer and also improved appearance of my saggy mummy tummy'.

Boots Expert Total Body Anti-Cellulite Cream

 6.21/10 A refreshing cream fomulation with an 'advanced formula', so Boots tell us, which includes antioxidants and vitamin E. (We also noted ginseng on the eye-challenging ingredients list.) After 28 days of use, 78 per cent of Boots' own testers saw an improvement in orange-peel – and it worked for some of our testers, too.

Testers say: 'Light, creamy lotion sank in immediately; overall tone

tip

● **Sip eight large glasses of still water daily.**
● **Eat plenty of veg, salads and protein (organic, where possible); avoid sugary foods, bread, pasta, rice, potatoes.**
● **Take moderate exercise daily: walking, swimming, stretching (yoga, etc), dancing.**
● **Dry skin brush daily before bathing/showering: we like Origins' lightweight Raffe Body Brush (under a tenner).**

of skin improved, and very soft and smooth – would like to try it with exercise, but would buy before a bikini holiday' • 'loved the smell – certainly a great body cream and may help cellulite with body brushing, exercise and weight loss' • 'skin less bumpy – firmer and smoother' • 'I think the massage definitely helps; skin tone slightly improved over six weeks, little bit tighter and smoother-looking' • 'easy: took a few minutes every evening; my lumpy, bumpy, wobbly thighs are now much smoother and firmer – and I lost an inch! Possibly down to the kneading action'.

L'Oréal Perfectslim Anti-Cellulite Gel-Cream

6/10 A gel-cream product with a silky, non-sticky finish; again, in L'Oréal's own tests on 101 women, dimpled skin appeared smoother and firmer

within four weeks. The key ingredient (which has a very L'Oréal-ish name) is Fibre-elastyl – a refining ingredient which is the result, they say, of five years' research. Again, list price is slightly over £10.

Testers say: 'Easy to do, and skin immediately smoother; after six weeks, texture of thighs much smoother and slightly firmer; also my upper arms – I loved this' • 'a great product, but will only work properly if you combine it with better diet, exercise and more water' • 'took a little time to be absorbed; after six weeks, definite improvement in skin texture' • 'skin slightly tighter – not quite as "moundy" – but I also lost some weight when testing' • 'less dimpling and size of dimples smaller; wobbly bits much firmer' • 'good clear instructions on massage application, with diagrams'.

face moves

Using good skincare products is vital, but how you apply them is just as important, says Geraldine Howard of Aromatherapy Associates: 'Simple facial massage can generate an enormous difference, helping to fade fine lines, slow down slackness, and make skin bright and glowing.'

Here are Geraldine's top tips for boosting your skincare with facial massage…

Mini face-lift Always work upwards, to give the facial tissue a gentle lift.

Rev up your cleanse Give your whole face a mini-treatment when you cleanse. Make lots of little, firm circling movements with your fingertips from jaw to hairline, to boost circulation, help remove impurities and generate radiant, healthy skin.

Smooth on moisturiser (any kind, including oils and serums) with your finger tips, working in alternate sweeping movements from your bosom up your neck and face to your hairline.

Bust jawline tension Your jaw holds stress, so it benefits from daily hands-on massage. With

your jaw clenched, rotate your fore and middle fingers quite hard from your chin up your jawline to the joint in front of your ears. Use a little facial oil to ease the routine. Then, using all fingertips, work up either side of the jawline, applying pressure to the bone, to firm the area.

Lift your cheekbones Do this by placing your fore and middle fingers either side of your nostrils at the base of your nose. Imagine you have a row of dots about 1cm apart just under your cheekbones, and apply pressure to each dot, working up to the hairline. Use a rose-based facial oil if possible, to further boost the circulation. Repeat morning and night, and during the day if you wish – it's fantastic for a quick lift before going out.

Open your eyes Help prevent fine lines around the eye area,

and smooth existing ones, by working from the outside of the eye in towards the nose. Dip your ring fingers in your eye product (or facial moisturiser), and draw them gently down the bone to the inner corner. To help drain any puffiness, lightly tap along the bone with your fingertips; extend across your whole face to invigorate it.

Banish that frown When applying a moisturiser or facial oil, massage out any frown lines with your fingertips, using an upwards and outwards motion. For vertical frown lines, place your middle fingers above the bridge of your nose, then work your fingers alternately up the lines. You can make quite quick but deep movements as you get practised. Not only does it help smooth lines, it's a fantastic way to relax your mind. Who needs expensive Botox jabs, now?

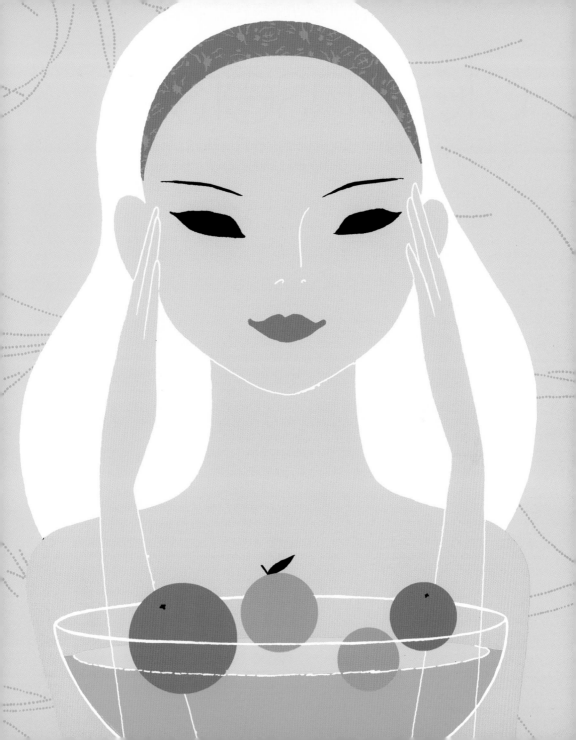

tried & tested
cleansers

This was a confusing category: two good products at SuperSteal prices – and a raft of others that came way, way down the score chart. So, because cleansing is such a vital skincare step, we've also listed three Tried & Tested products we swear by (see 'we love', opposite), which cost a tad over our 'beauty steal' ceiling for full size – but all supply 30ml sample/travel sizes for under a fiver.

 Neutrogena Visibly Clear 2-in-1 Wash Mask

8.1/10 We've never before encountered a cleanser which can double as a mask, as this promises: use daily as a wash, or leave on to deep-cleanse pores. Testers liked its packaging. **Testers say:** 'Simple to use and effective at controlling my spots without drying' • 'removed make-up easily, but you need an eye make-up remover too' • 'as good as my more expensive cleanser' • 'good creamy texture that spread easily' • 'a little goes a long way, so it's cost effective'.

 The Body Shop Nutriganics™ Foaming Facial Wash ✿

7.95/10 There are two reasons we're pleased to see this new entry from the Body Shop:

it's always good to be able to recommend a foaming cleanser, and it's from a range that's their first foray into (Ecocert-certified) organic skincare, with Community Traded babassu oil from Brazil. Testers found it didn't remove eye make-up/mascara, though. **Testers say:** 'Ten out of ten for this luxurious-feeling thick foam which you put on dry skin; far better than my current foaming cleanser – removed make-up easily, but needed a separate eye make-up remover' • 'no need for toner, owing to rinsing off, and skin felt fresh after' • 'removed my foundation effortlessly; not so good with eye make-up' • 'I would happily use this, but it's functional, rather than a treat' • 'easy-to-use pump-action bottle; one pump enough for face' • 'also really good for shaving legs!'.

 Skin Blossom Organic Bloom Gentle Cleansing Milk ✿✿

7.39/10 A finalist in the 2009 Soil Association Organic Beauty Awards, this 88 per cent organic cleansing milk is vegan, free from artificial fragrance, colour and petrochemicals, and gets its make-up melting power from sweet almond oil, glycerine and aloe vera.

Testers say: 'Easy to use; silky texture that spread smoothly; removed some mascara, but not all brands; skin lightly moisturised' • 'rather "amateur" packaging, but if I'd blind-tested it I would have been very satisfied' • 'didn't need a toner – and no make-up on my pillow!' • 'not greasy; face soft and silky; no tightness and lovely glow – could do with a better dispenser'.

we love

Given the choice, we'd always pay a wee bit more and go for one of these cleansers, two of which are certified organic – with the first one here being the Beauty Bible's highest-scoring cleanser ever!

Liz Earle Naturally Active Skincare Cleanse & Polish Hot Cloth Cleanser ✿

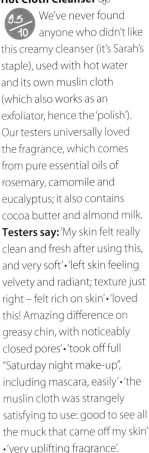

9.5/10 We've never found anyone who didn't like this creamy cleanser (it's Sarah's staple), used with hot water and its own muslin cloth (which also works as an exfoliator, hence the 'polish'). Our testers universally loved the fragrance, which comes from pure essential oils of rosemary, camomile and eucalyptus; it also contains cocoa butter and almond milk.

Testers say: 'My skin felt really clean and fresh after using this, and very soft' • 'left skin feeling velvety and radiant; texture just right – felt rich on skin' • 'loved this! Amazing difference on greasy chin, with noticeably closed pores' • 'took off full "Saturday night make-up", including mascara, easily' • 'the muslin cloth was strangely satisfying to use: good to see all the muck that came off my skin' • 'very uplifting fragrance'.

Essential Care Creamy Coconut Cleanser ✿ ✿ ✿

7.31/10 You can get a 30ml size of this for under a tenner to try it. Essential Care – a Soil Association-certified mother-and-daughter brand – recommend this for normal to dry or mature skins, with its skin-conditioning coconut and olive oils; remove with pads, or swish away with water.

Testers say: 'Lovely creamy texture that smoothed on easily and evenly with a good, old-fashioned quality; very good at removing even heavy eye make-up' • 'good product, especially if ethics is top of your list' • 'ten out of ten! Even better than the Beauty Bible's top-scoring cleanser, which I have used for years – did the job without irritating my sensitive skin. I will use it for ever' • 'perfect consistency, rich texture: subtle fragance (not very "coconutty"!). Greatly outperforms my usual cleanser'.

Essential Care Lemon & Tea Tree Facial Wash ✿ ✿ ✿

7.31/10 Scoring just less than the other Essential Care product (left), this, too, is available in a 30ml introductory/travel size. This mild, antiseptic rinse-off cleanser, infused with calming lavender and antibacterial tea tree, is targeted at normal-to-oily or acne-prone skins (though it didn't suit all of our spotty testers).

Testers say: 'Very easy to use; glided on easily; felt light and smelt clean and refreshing; removed light make-up effectively; skin felt nice and clean after; no toner necessary' • 'took off most make-up well, but not waterproof mascara' • 'left skin moisturised and well balanced' • 'says to avoid eyes but it didn't sting when it got in them' • 'skin was definitely not dry, but nicely cleansed without feeling stripped or tight; despite loving my usual cleanser, I'm still using this'.

tried & tested
cleansing wipes

Wipes are rapidly climbing the cleanser bestseller charts: it's sooo easy to swipe away the day before bedtime. All the options here have low price tags – but you'll actually get much better value from a balm-style, last-for-ages cleanser, used with a washable, longlasting muslin cloth, so we haven't awarded any SuperSteals. Still, if the alternative is falling into bed with your face on, they're a godsend. NB: testers say, do close the packet completely to avoid wipes drying out.

Nivea Visage Refreshing Facial Cleansing Wipes

8.2/10 This first featured in an earlier Beauty Bible, and we've included it because none of the two dozen wipe products we tested for this new book did better. They're alcohol free, and so non-drying – even though they're targeted at normal and combination skins. The fleecy texture features 'micro-sponges' to lift off gunk and grime.
Testers say: 'Ideal for daily use and compact enough for travelling'•'a few wipes removed mascara miraculously; convenient, effective and toning'•'wonderful to freshen up with this on a sticky day'•'particularly soft around the eyes'•'less "wet" than most wipes, but efficient, and not at all drying'.

Garnier Clean-Sensitive Velvety Smooth Anti-Tightness Wipes

7.9/10 'Anti-tightness' is a big selling point for wipes, because many women are put off by the alcohol in some, which really strips skin. These have a very gentle texture, and feature in a Garnier sub-range targeted at touchy skins.
Testers say: 'Very effective at cleaning; didn't have to rub, just swipe a wipe! Skin felt fine, not greasy or dry, just comfortable: didn't inflame my sensitive skin at all'•'wipes came out individually from easy-to-reseal packaging'•'took off full make-up, though I had to use slight pressure to remove mascara'•'removed make-up efficiently and quickly; skin felt fresh and clean, but not tight'•'the best I have used; cooling and cleansing'•'skin was

we love

squeaky clean; the opening never lost its stickiness, unlike most packets; great to take on holiday or for nights away'.

L'Oreal Demaq Expert Rich, Ultra Effective Make-up Removing Cloths

 7.71/10 This range from L'Oréal – a new entry here – is designed to remove even the heaviest professional make-up (even eye make-up), with more concentrated ingredients than the brand's other wipes. A couple of testers found the pack's plastic seal to be a bit fragile.

Testers say: 'Was very impressed: took off tinted sunblock and eye make-up with a couple of swipes; skin felt smooth and moisturised after; excellent packaging' • 'far better than any wipes I've tried before: impressed by how easily they removed make-up and the convenience; no reason to fall asleep with my face on now!' • 'generous-sized cloths, which felt good quality and thick; great to travel with, or if I'm feeling lazy' • 'skin felt perfect after, not too dry – would definitely treat myself to them' • 'very efficient at removing make-up, even mascara' • 'loved the plastic flip lid, which stopped wipes drying out; really did the

> Jo doesn't really go in for cleansing wipes, except in true beauty emergencies, when she opts for **Skin Therapy 4 in 1 Facial Wipes** (exclusive to Sainsbury's), which don't have the overpowering fragrance of some others, and at a pinch can remove eye make-up, too. Sarah really does love having them in her bag for train travel and staying overnight: she opts for **Faith in Nature 3-in-1 Facial Wipes**, which are 100 per cent natural and biodegradable, and infused with organic aloe vera, allantoin and vitamin C.

job well – great for a quick fix. Definitely my facial wipe of choice now'.

Skin Wisdom Daily Care 4 in 1 Cleansing Wipes

 7.7/10 Golly, can a mere cleansing wipe really pack four actions into one sheet? Cleansing, toning, moisturising (though we'd always recommend applying your usual moisturiser after cleansing), and budging eye make-up, too (even waterproof), so they promise. Skin-friendly ingredients in this Tesco offering include green tea, camomile and shea butter.

Testers say: 'Ten out of ten for fuss-free product with great results; great for the gym; fits in my bag, and I like that I can wipe my face and it doesn't feel like dried prune; I will buy' • 'lovely fresh smell, good packaging; skin

felt clean and refreshed with no stickiness' • 'no problems removing make-up, though did need eye make-up remover for mascara' • 'I use these every day – the best I've found. No gritty or sore eyes and great price'.

Botanics Quick Fix Cleansing Wipes

7.7/10 With mallow extract to calm skin plus other plant ingredients, these marry botanicals (from sustainable sources) with skincare high-tech and are suitable for sensitive complexions, say Boots, although one tester found them drying.

Testers say: 'Very efficient; packaging good, and nice fragrance' • 'my skin felt clean, but quite dry' • 'easy to carry around' • 'removed eye make-up well' • 'excellent – large wipe left skin comfortable and clean'.

tried & tested
toners

If you really want to save money, we always advise you can skip this step in your beauty regime. But plenty of women simply don't feel fresh faced without a swipe of toner – so here are the top-performing affordable choices. (Which, in some cases, did better than many products at five or even ten times the price.)

 Botanics Organic Rosewater Toner ❀❀

 A little touch of glycerine has been added to this simple, Damask rosewater toner, for its 'humectant' properties (ie, it helps attract water to the skin). All the ingredients are certified organic, Boots claim, but the product hasn't been independently audited by a third-party organic certifier – that's why we've given it only two daisies for naturalness, not three. It did get some very high scores. **Testers say:** 'Lovely fragrance, and I really enjoyed using this,

despite the unsophisticated packaging! My skin felt velvety soft, refreshed and hydrated and it removed all final traces of make-up; excellent' • 'moisturiser seemed to glide on skin afterwards' • 'cooling and toning, with no tightness; can also be used as a cologne, and reduced itching and redness on my legs! A very comforting product' • 'very refreshing and hydrating' • 'nice product that does the job'.

The Body Shop Aloe Calming Toner

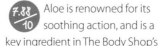 Aloe is renowned for its soothing action, and is a key ingredient in The Body Shop's

sensitive-skin range. Here, a lightweight toner in a flip-top bottle (which makes it more economical to use than some of the other toner options here that have wider necks, making it easy to over-drench your cotton pad). **Testers say:** 'I never use toner but this is such a pleasure that it's converted a long-term toner hater! Particularly gorgeous for the summer, and when travelling' • 'nice fresh texture and smell and didn't make my dry sensitive skin feel tight at all' • 'cooling and calming; very pleasant, and felt it was soothing my skin as well as removing last traces of make-up' • 'moisturiser sank in well after using this'.

Neal's Yard Remedies Rosewater ❀❀

 The product we prefer ourselves, in this category: a blissful rosewater – with a touch of aloe vera and glycerine, again to boost the skin-quenching properties of the skin-freshener. For some reason, Neal's Yard has 'self-certified' this organic product (rather than used Ecocert or the Soil Association), so we only award two daisies for naturalness. (We know Neal's Yard uphold the very highest standards, but we are still keen that products which claim to be organic seek external verification – it's the only way to stop all the bandwagoning that goes on.)

Testers say: 'Lovely rose-based fragrance; skin felt refreshed and fully cleansed, but not too tight; no stinging; moisturiser sank in well' • 'very soothing and delicious; lovely cooling sensation for the skin – if you're a toner addict, this is the one for you!' • 'love the packaging – simple, functional and stylish, though not practical to travel with, as it's glass: I liked the feel on my skin and it seemed to prepare it for moisturiser' • 'my skin felt instantly hydrated, slightly tighter, extremely clean and had a beautiful scent' • 'such a traditional cosmetic, but still works wonders on modern-day stressed-out skin'.

Weleda Iris Facial Toner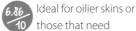

 6.86/10 Ideal for oilier skins or those that need balancing, this contains a touch of alcohol as well as toning witch hazel and lemon. (This is the only

---

tip

Toner – especially if kept in the fridge – can be good for waking up skin. But we like this tip from our friend Marcia Kilgore, genius founder of Soap & Glory (and fab FitFlops): 'When you want to wake up fast and fake an energised glow, dunk your face into a sink of ice-cold water,' she advises.

---

toner with alcohol in that our testers rated.) It helps restore the skin's acid/alkali balance without drying, though, because the key ingredient – iris – helps store and regulate moisture in the skin. We rather love the fact that Weleda resist snazzy redesigns and have kept the simple blue bottle for almost-ever.

Testers say: 'Pure, fresh, comforting fragrance; skin felt refreshed and soft; I've used many that left my skin screaming for moisturiser, but this one is gentle, delicate and reviving; people complimented me on how lovely my skin looked, and it can only be down to this

---

wonderful toner' • 'I have little mobility in my hands but this was easy to open/dispense, etc; skin felt squeaky clean and looked clearer' • 'left skin lovely and cool; made me feel brighter and more awake in the morning' • 'I was impressed with this product: very pleasant to use; made skin feel fresh and clean'.

 Skin Wisdom Daily Care Refreshing Toner

 6.7/10 In this super-affordable option from Tesco's basic skincare range (which is formulated with Bharti Vyas, the well-known Ayurvedic facialist), green tea blends with soothing camomile and toning, refreshing witch hazel.

Testers say: 'As good as the more expensive one I usually use, and much cheaper: skin felt refreshed and hydrated' • 'my skin felt very clean; either I wasn't taking all my make-up off before, or this sloughed off some dead skin cells; a couple of times my skin tingled, but then it calmed down; it gave my skin a polish' • 'felt like it "sealed" my skin – moisturiser seemed to soak in more quickly' • 'my skin felt completely refreshed and clean; didn't dry my skin like other toners – a pleasant experience'.

tried & tested
concealers

Concealer is a 'hallelujah' product: we're eternally grateful it exists, to magic away dark circles, shadows, blemishes, red veins (always on top of foundation). These concealers scored a little lower than YSL's classic Touche Eclat – with its almost unassailable score of 9.33 out of ten – (though one tester vows she's found a rival) but they also lag way behind, pricewise: definite steals for fast flawlessness.

Maybelline Pure Minerals Concealer

 A stellar performance (several '10s') for this new entry sends it rocketing to the top of the concealer charts. Although the 'minerals' tag is a bit hype-y (the mineral titanium dioxide is a key ingredient in most concealers), this lightweight option does have all the luminous light-reflective powers associated with mineral make-up, especially good for covering up dark shadows.

Testers say: 'Very easy to blend in with fingers; very good on dark circles and small blemishes;

not drying and looked very natural in all lighting: compares well to my usual, much more expensive concealer' • 'covered thread veins, small scars, dark circles well – blemishes very well; I used the sponge applicator which was very easy, I loved this product: it gave brilliant coverage and completely hid dark marks from recent spots, but didn't look as if I was wearing much make-up' • 'the best I've found; covered well, didn't crease' • 'absolutely brilliant, especially on uneven pigmentation: I used a concealer brush and it worked wonderfully with my expensive foundations and blushers' • 'at last, something which hides my dark shadows and doesn't cake in my wrinkles!'.

GOSH Touch-up Concealer

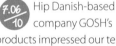 Hip Danish-based company GOSH's products impressed our testers. This concealer features a teensy

---

tip

'Save your concealer for last: it adds a polish to the entire face. When I started out, I dotted on a peach-tone concealer to actress Lara Flynn Boyle's face and it acted like an eraser – getting rid of any under-eye tones.' Sue Devitt

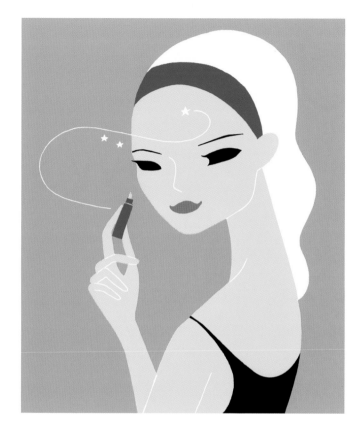

Testers say: 'I was surprised and delighted that something so cheap could hold its own – it's great at covering dark circles, though not so good for thread veins – but for the price…?!'• 'blends extremely easily; covered marks and scars well, and lightened dark areas'•'modern sassy packaging'•'top marks for covering up dried-up flaky spots!'.

The Body Shop Flawless Skin Perfecting Concealer

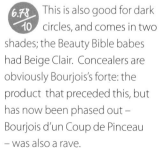 **6.5/10** A sassy, sexy little twist-up silver stick of concealer (so glam, frankly, you could get away with disguising your flaws in public!), this comes in four shades (our testers tried one of the darker tones, 03), and is enriched with boabab oil and zinc oxide, to combat impurities. The 'active essence' can be seen in the product core, but it blends on skin contact.

Testers say: 'Blended in easily once it had warmed up slightly; covered small scars brilliantly; stayed fresh looking all day – a wonder product'•'some days I didn't even need to use foundation; I never want to be without this'•'nice neat little applicator'•'I don't often use concealers but I love this; quick, easy and looks very natural'.

brush inside the cap for precision application. (You can also use it as a plumping lip base, in the lightest shade – 1 – which we trialled.) Perfume free, too.

Testers say: 'Covered thread veins and pigmentation well; not so good on spots. I was very pleased, and loved the soft brush' •'quite thin consistency, so blended well; brush made it easy to apply'•'didn't cake at all, once I got the hang of it'•'creamy, not gloopy, and didn't cake; good for dark under-eye shadows'.

Bourjois Brush Concealer

6.78/10 This is also good for dark circles, and comes in two shades; the Beauty Bible babes had Beige Clair. Concealers are obviously Bourjois's forte: the product that preceded this, but has now been phased out – Bourjois d'un Coup de Pinceau – was also a rave.

tried & tested
powder eyeshadows

We'll be honest: we've rather been eyeshadow 'snobs', devoted to our Bobbi Brown and Chanel shadows (with a bit of M.A.C. thrown in). But these high-scoring products – which outperformed many much pricier rivals – have made us have a rethink, and we've also found some favourites of our own. We were probably prejudiced by early encounters with gritty, grainy, garish eyeshadows. By contrast, testers praised this selection for smooth application, texture and staying power. With results like these, it really is a case of 'why pay more?'.

Prestige Skin Loving Minerals Dramatic Minerals Eyeshadow

8.52/10 An amazing score for Prestige's mineral-based shadow, which, like all its make-up, is 100 per cent oil free, talc free and paraben free, but enriched with ingredients such as shea butter, camomile and antioxidant vitamins to deliver skin benefits. The stylish Perspex palette flips open to reveal a soft-pressed powder. Several shades did well, but 03 Citrine, a soft, yellowy green, got top score.

Testers say: 'Ten out of ten for this easy-to-apply, creamy, slightly shimmery powder shadow; I used a brush but fingers do fine; much better than any other I've used' • 'the best I've used: the price is a bonus!' • 'even colour, easy to build up' • 'loved it – but the packaging was flimsy'.

Myface Eye Touch Eye Shadow

8.11/10 We love make-up artist Charlotte Tilbury's Myface make-up range – and our testers really rated this eyeshadow trio, with nifty packaging and textures soft and smooth enough to satisfy the very demanding Charlotte. Most of her range is divvied up into fair, medium or dark skintones, but her philosophy is that, once those basics are right, you can get away with any colour shadow. Our testers were sent a trio of wearable browns, Morocco 3, which features a

we love

glitzy 'Blingtone' shade, with a foil-effect metallic finish in gold. **Testers say:** 'Lovely natural shades that were a doddle to apply: could achieve a natural day or more dramatic evening look. Incredibly smooth and velvety soft; didn't have the feeling of being over-made-up and didn't affect my sensitive eyes' • 'pure delight to use' • 'well thought out, from packaging and applicator to the great shades' • 'great "bling" shade to use over the other two' • 'gave a very sophisticated "neutral" eye, with a subtle glimmer twist' • 'very glam finished effect' • 'small enough to pop in your bag, and longlasting'.

Bourjois Little Round Pot Eyeshadow

 With the same domed shape and soft texture as their blusher, these little pots of colour from Bourjois in ten shades (we trialled 54 Marron Glacé, a bronze shimmer) are beauty classics. Use with a slightly damp brush, as they suggest, for more depth of colour and shimmer.
Testers say: 'Fabulously easy to use; dinky portable little pot with a great firm catch. I liked using it damp. It's shimmery, but not too

> **Sarah has discovered the amazing Bourjois single palette range, (with useful-sized mirror and proper-ish brush) called Ombre Stretch, which comes in a range of good colours, including Gold Definition, Extreme White and bronzey Flexible Brown, plus the fabulous Brun Nylon (see page 89). And in Jo's bag, you'll find the Bourjois Little Round Pot Eyeshadow and the Myface Eye Touch palettes that our testers also considered award-worthy.**

glitzy for daywear' • 'a revelation; I've missed out on eyeshadow until now – thanks, Beauty Bible' • 'very smooth, easily blended shadow with a slight gold shimmer, on a par with my more expensive brand, and stayed put nearly all day' • 'everything I need in an eyeshadow'.

  e.l.f. Brightening Eye Color
e.l.f. products are so affordable you'll have to pinch yourself – yet this is as smooth as products five times the price. Nine compacts to choose from – and we were sent Butternut, a very wearable combo of four neutrals, from mid-beige to smoky brown.
Testers say: 'Compared very well with my much more expensive palette; stayed on well and needed very little touching up for evening; colour range gave a

very good effect – and I received a number of compliments' • 'exceptional value and good quality; a great way for my teenage daughter to experiment, too' • 'packaging looked quite cheap but the colour went on very well – better than some expensive brands' • 'lovely effect; colour was even and the contrast created the perfect smoky-eye look' • 'really liked this, and the four shades, so you have a day and evening look in one palette'.

  W7 Eyeshadow
W7 is named after the London postcode where they started, with the aim of 'producing the best possible cosmetics for the lowest possible price'. They cover the full colour spectrum: eccentric shades for teens and classic tones 'for the more

mature woman looking for a cheap treat' (!) – which, we guess, includes the wearable brown shade of powder shadow, 12 Rosewood, which nine of our testers enjoyed.

Testers say: 'Slight shimmer wasn't too much for day, and could be boosted for evening with a loose shimmer powder on top' • 'nice colour; looked like I'd made an effort, without looking overdone' • 'cute compact with teeny mirror' • 'good finished effect: nice colour that would suit most people and lasted throughout the day' • 'a decent smooth powder, faded to a paler hue with a subtle glimmer; very portable and usable compact'.

GOSH Quattro Eyeshadow

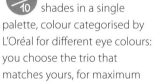 Danish brand GOSH submitted a couple of palettes in different shades. Despite having been sent to two different panels, they scored within a micro-point of each other – with the silver-based Platinum palette squeaking in just ahead of Driftwood, a quad of browns.

Testers say: 'Some of the best eyeshadows I've ever used – loved the intensity of the colours and the shimmery, smoky finish' • 'I thought the shades would be

Best results come, our testers found, if you blend, blend, blend with a good brush – see page 8 for more.

too young for me, but looked trendy and professional; smooth, easy application, stayed put well – and caused no problem with my contact lenses' • 'lovely colour combinations and attractive packaging' • 'great cheap alternative for everyday use'.

L'Oréal Color Appeal Trio Pro

Three smooth powder shades in a single palette, colour categorised by L'Oréal for different eye colours: you choose the trio that matches yours, for maximum eye enhancement. The palette our testers rated was for blue eyes, containing bone, caramel and taupe shades.

Testers say: 'Finished effect was glamorous, and staying power pretty impressive' • 'excellent for a cheaper-end shadow; no crepey eye effect on my older eyelids; worked as well as the expensive shadows I usually wear' • 'a strong

evening look which really brought out my eyes' • 'bit sparkly for work, but would work well for non-work days, particularly sunny ones'.

 e.l.f. Mineral Eyeshadow ❀ ❀

Clever little e.l.f., with two award-winners here: this is a 100 per cent mineral eyeshadow in loose powder format, which is also a top 'steal' for our green/natural readers. It comes in 18 shades; for some reason the name given to the goldy/taupe we sent to our testers is 'Celebrity'.

Testers say: 'Very impressed: a nice product with no-nonsense packaging; blending reduced the sparkle to a shimmer – I'm 52 and sparkly eyeshadow is a no-no!' • 'gave shimmery, gorgeous eyes, and no irritation, even with my contact lenses' • 'good value, and I would recommend it to friends, which says a lot' • 'this was great as a shimmery highlighter' • 'very easy to use: tap some of the powder in the lid, dip in a brush and then apply; lovely smooth, silky consistency; loved the colour, which is ideal for parties; I was pleased that it contained 100 per cent natural minerals with nothing else added – made me feel my skin would approve'.

Cream eyeshadows

There weren't such spectacularly good results for cream-formula eyeshadows as for powder ones – in fact, only one contender (right) remains worthy of a mention among the 15 or so we trialled – but this steal was a real eye-opener (sorry!) for some testers.

 we love

There are precious few creamy eyeshadows at an affordable price which float our boat. However, Jo is keen both on the Rimmel product (right), and also Maybelline's somewhat similar, light-as-air Dream Mousse Eyecolour (despite the fact it didn't 'wow' our testers), which can be swiped on with a finger. The most wearable shades, she finds, are Caramel Karma and Suede Sensation.

 Rimmel Colour Mousse Eyeshadow 8 Hour

 Rimmel submitted this for testing in lots of different shades from the eight on offer. And, despite being sent to different teams up and down the country, the scores came in within a fraction of each other. These little pots of eye colour contain 25 per cent purified water, so they have a

tip

Many cheap cream shadows crease faster than a linen suit, so prep your lids by using a little loose powder or neutral powder shadow underneath. Or take a dry make-up sponge and press lightly on to the lid after eyeshadow, so it soaks up any extra oil but leaves the colour.

refreshing action on the skin. They are easily blendable with a finger, and Rimmel promise they last up to eight hours; 005 Glitz – a suits-everyone creamy-beige – romped home slightly ahead of 004 Splash, a powdery blue.

Testers say: 'Easy to use with fingers or own brush – no applicator; both ways work; looks very shimmery but that blends in as you brush, so you can choose how you want it'•'as light as the proverbial feather and doesn't drag at all; a subtle wash of colour that you can build up to something more dramatic; it's GREAT, and at least half the price of my usual ones' •'gave subtle definition to my eyes and lasted from 8am into the late afternoon, as promised; then I reapplied, and no caking – great'• 'texture was just like a real mousse and didn't crease at all'•'I love the texture and staying power – once I'd practised a bit!'.

tried & tested
eyelash curlers

For some women these are a must-have, and for others they are a total waste of space in a make-up kit (or just make you feel very peculiar, like Sarah). For those who can't live without them, however, here goes…

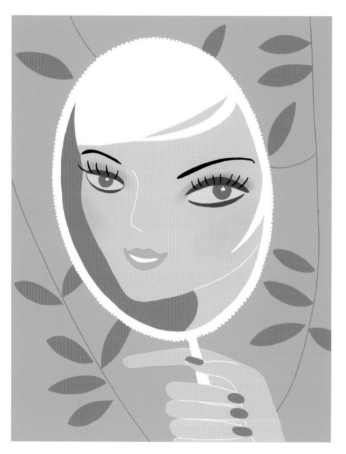

Tweezerman Eyelash Curler

7.88/10 Officially, this isn't a 'steal' (the list price is over a tenner). But at websites like the reputable HQhair.com – one of our 'Beauty Bible-approved' sites – you can find it for less than that. In general, you have to be careful with buying beauty on the internet: products can be sourced via what's known as the 'grey' market, meaning stock can be out of date or discontinued. (That's why at www.beautybible.com we carefully screen the sites we approve, to avoid that.) But with a metal product like an eyelash curler, there's really no problem buying online, especially if you can get it for less! Tweezerman have an incredibly high reputation for their make-up accessories, which are often quoted as 'celebrity must-haves'. Tweezerman offer replacement

tip

To enhance the eye-opening power of your eyelash curlers, you can blast with a hair-dryer on hot for five seconds (no more) before using, to mimic the effect of the (pricier) heated ones now on the market.

rubber tips for these curlers, which have a 'scissor' grip.

Testers say: 'Very easy instructions; took a maximum of ten seconds to curl my lashes; a huge improvement on my others' • 'gave a soft, natural curl, not a "crimped" look' • 'made my eyes look more wide awake and slightly brighter' • 'these are amazing and don't even need heating; they seem more expensive than other metal curlers because there is a soft, cushioned feel when you squeeze the handles together'.

Red by Kiss Perfect Curl Deluxe Eyelash Curler

7.10/10 These salon-quality curlers have a 'spring' design, 'to provide the ideal tension for the perfect curl'. They also feature rubberised finger grips, delivering a non-slip surface to the handle, for better control. The pad is silicone (most

are rubber), which is said to be more flexible – again, for curl-boosting reasons. There's a spare pad for the curler, which we suggest you put in A VERY SAFE PLACE as it's eminently loseable.

Testers say: 'Very easy-to-use instructions and design; applicator was comfy to hold and easy to press down; pads felt spongy and not too hard against my lashes, but still gave good effect' • 'lashes looked longer and eyes opened; combined with mascara, my eyes "popped" much more' • 'eyelash curlers have a new-found place in my make-up routine; easy to use, even for a novice; lashes looked a fair bit longer and eyes wider and brighter; curl lasted all day' • 'well designed, with nice handle; gave a nice even curl, and didn't tear out lashes' • 'more comfy than my Shu Uemura ones and almost as good, so would buy'.

Revlon Eyelash Curler

 6.33/10 We're incredibly impressed with the Revlon range of accessories, which launched fairly recently, and our testers certainly liked these curlers, in a sleek design that fits close to the lash line, for maximum curl. Unlike most curlers, Revlon maintain that these can be used on mascara-ed lashes as well as bare lashes (which is the general rule).

Testers say: 'Ten out of ten! Amazing' • 'curl lasted when set with mascara – which seems to apply to all eyelash curlers' • 'very simple and easy to use; comfortable, too; curl enhanced my eye; lashes definitely looked longer, and with mascara I can achieve a long flirty-lash look' • 'I have used cheap and expensive curlers and these came pretty high up in terms of ease of use: sometimes I catch my skin or get a clamp mark on the lashes, but neither happened with the Revlon Curler, which I was very pleased with' • 'you only need to hold them in place for five seconds, so quite comfortable; make a huge impact on wideness of eyes; good that they come with a spare pad'.

tried & tested
eyeliners

Wow! The top-scoring pencils here did better in our trials than almost all the big (more expensive) brands that we sent out at the same time – so they're not just best buys (in fact, almost all SuperSteals), but best bets all round.

 Barbara Daly Make-up for Tesco Eye Pencil

8.36/10 The products that legendary make-up pro Barbara created for this line raised the bar for own-label beauty ranges in the supermarket world, and are as good as ever (although she is 'divorced' from them now). Testers gave a stellar score to this soft-textured pencil, which glides over the lid without dragging. In four shades: we dispatched Dark Brown to our panel of ten. **Testers say:** 'Ten out of ten for this amazing product; brilliant to sharpen, lovely to use, slightly smudgeable – I would buy!' • 'I was delighted at how easily I could draw a line without pressing hard; could use for a fine or a heavy line – a joy to use' • 'easy to get a defined line or a nice smoky effect' • 'smooth, with great staying power; beautiful deepish brown, with no sign of ginger – Barbara Daly is such a clever lady'.

 Collection 2000 Glam Crystals Dazzling Gel Liner

 7.42/10 Something quite different, with this product: a somewhat disco-glam gel liner, with its own brush, that's perfect for a bold after-dark look. It slicks along the lid, adding a liquid line of silver/gold. A quirky entry, but testers loved it.

Testers say: 'Very easy and straightforward to apply; you could draw a thin or thicker line – really liked it; lovely colour, though not for everyday!' • 'fun product, clear gel with a dense amount of gold glitter particles, which is flattering to my fair skintone – great value for money' • 'nice soft brush; easy to apply precisely; you could smudge if you did it immediately' • 'I thought, "Help! I'm too old to wear that outside the house", but you could make it really subtle – my 24-year-old daughter loved it, too, using a much stronger line' • 'this product lasts well and comes off easily with make-up remover'.

♡ we love

Jo generally uses a very smudgy eyeliner pencil by Sue Devitt which is generally well above the £10 mark, but after-dark also likes the hippy-chick smokiness of L'Oréal Kohl Minerals Powder Liner, a sponge-tipped wand that you 'dip' into the powder liner. Sarah's wedded to GOSH eyeliner pencils (right under her lower lashes) for their amazing value and performance.

tip

You arrive on holiday – but your make-up doesn't... At an absolute pinch, you can carefully use a burnt match gently stroked along the lash-line to create a smoky, rock-chick eye look. (Only for a beauty SOS: it's clearly not ophthalmologically or dermatologically tested – but it's one of those little tricks that does actually work.)

Revlon Luxurious Color™ Eyeliner

7.37/10 The velvety texture of this pencil – with deep pigments for intense colour – has an 'extra soft built-in tip applicator', they explain, for precise application. Six shades, including Antiqued Gold and Brushed Pewter (good for evenings), but our testers were seduced by the less daring Black Velvet.

Testers say: 'I'm terrible at applying eyeliner but this is the easiest ever – I will be wearing eyeliner more often now – so thank you!' • 'soft, felt-tip-type texture made it easy to apply; with practice, I managed a fine line – very handy to take around; impressed by longevity' • 'very smudgeable if you wanted, but set quite firmly after a few minutes, so you don't get a panda-eye effect' • 'I'm blonde so prefer brown liner, but this is much nicer than most black liners'.

 Prestige Waterproof Automatic Eyeliner

7.25/10 One for the beach, this, from US brand Prestige, who've done awfully well in the make-up categories for Beauty Steals. We like 'automatic' eyeliners: they twist up (so never need sharpening, and won't ever become a stub that scratches the eye skin). Useful to have a waterproof option in this category, for sweaty days and holidays, and it comes in nine shades. Some testers raved about this, while others couldn't get to grips.

Testers say: 'Eyeliner has always been hit and miss for me, until now: this is so easy to use, I could draw a perfect line every time – love it!' • 'good everyday eye pencil – great for the handbag; more of a relaxed line than precise, so pretty smudgeable' • 'I really, really like this pencil: it was very easy to apply, gave a good line and smudged easily – very soft to put on and didn't make my eyes sting or water'.

tried & tested
eye make-up removers

We weren't sure what we'd find in this category: would cheap eye make-up removers irritate testers' eyes? Would they swipe away mascara (the biggest challenge) without rubbing? Would they smell as cheap as they really are? Here are the eye-opening results.

 Nivea Visage Extra-Gentle Eye Make-Up Remover Lotion

 This lotion is light, non-greasy, non-irritant, ophthalmologically tested and even suitable for contact lens wearers; Nivea promise us that it 'removes all traces of make-up while retaining precious moisture around the delicate eye area'. Our testers agreed.

Testers say: 'Couldn't be easier to use: no effort – just a couple of gentle strokes needed to remove make-up and mascara; I have to be really careful with my sensitive eyes but this was the gentlest product I've tried' • 'fantastic product; felt good to use, caused no irritation and did the job – has changed my mind about eye make-up removers, which I never used before' • 'this product took a matter of seconds to remove mascara, eye shadow and base – though it struggled with long-life lipstick' • 'as a contact lens wearer, I found this to be very gentle'.

 tip

Bothered by specks and flecks and smudges that give you panda eyes by the end of the day? No need to completely re-do your eye-make-up: Smudgees are genius Q-tip style wands impregnated with remover, which are great for cleaning up smudges and specks, at any time (see **DIRECTORY**).

Simple Eye Make-up Remover

7.66/10 Simple's USP is that, like Clinique, their products are great for the sensitive-skinned – and, in this case, for the sensitive-eyed: again, this is said to be fine for contact lens wearers, and also features pro-vitamin B5, to condition and soften the fragile skin in the eye zone.

Testers say: 'Ten out of ten for this – really easy, gentle and fragrance free; did the job and for the price it's amazing – and not greasy like the expensive product I've been using for years' • 'no stinging or redness on my extremely sensitive eyes – a pleasure to use, and removed most eye make-up quickly and easily; a little more effort for mascara' • 'I'm a lens wearer but this didn't upset my eyes at all; easily removed all make-up – very light around the eye area; other products have given me little white spots'.

The Body Shop Camomile Gentle Eye Make-up Remover

7.22/10 This is one of The Body Shop's 'classic' products, which has been in the range virtually since the year dot: a gentle, soothing and cooling lotion featuring an element from camomile which is known for its calming action, as well as the humectant glycerine – so it's completely non-drying.

Testers say: 'Worked like a charm; contained at least some natural ingredients and is an absolute steal!' • 'made a fair whack at everything except my Chanel Inimitable waterproof mascara, which practically needs a palette knife to get off!' • 'very favourably impressed by this gentle formula' • 'no soreness or sensitivity; took off every trace of eye make-up, with a little extra persuasion on the waterproof mascara – I would definitely buy it'.

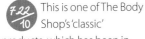

Jo is hugely impressed by the Skin Therapy Eye Make-up Remover Pads: soft and gentle, effective even on mascara, in a packet of 25 wipes that you can throw in your suitcase (to minimise leakage risks) while travelling.

Botanics Soothing Eye Make-up Remover ❋

6.87/10 This Boots range incorporates active plant extracts (and is authenticated by the Royal Botanic Gardens, Kew); the key plant element here is an Icelandic moss with a high sugar content, which helps to hydrate and calm skin while cleansing. It's a bi-phase product, which means that it needs to be shaken vigorously to intermix the oil and lotion. (NB: two of our testers reported that they found their eyes stung after using this product, but several others gave it high marks, so we have left it in.)

Testers say: 'Amazingly effective; didn't leave a residue, so you can put on make-up immediately if you want. I've always had to go high end for eye make-up remover, so this is a pleasant surprise' • 'very easy, as long as I remembered to shake the bottle hard to mix' • 'easy and effective, but too greasy for lens wearers' • 'very gentle and very effective, but very oily' • 'removed waterproof mascara easily, but the eye area needed freshening afterwards to get rid of the oil'.

tried & tested
treats for tired eyes

We get more questions about how to tackle under-eye baggage and dark circles at www.beautybible.com than we do about any other beauty woe. The answer's a mixture of lifestyle tips – see our website Q&A – and effective products. And we've found some good ones, at eye-poppingly low prices.

Green People Eye Gel ✿✿

7.07/10 The top scorer here is all natural, with plant proteins to reduce puffiness, along with fair-traded Roman camomile. Though our testers didn't trial this for long-term benefits, Green People now incorporate two anti-ageing botanicals – *Caesalpinia spinosa* (spiny holdback bush) and an edible seaweed. A great tip is to mix a tiny amount of the gel into your foundation, to firm the area and help make-up stay in place.

Testers say: 'Instant, very refreshing, cooling effect from this rich gel: skin feels tighter' • 'ten out of ten: easy to pat around the orbital bone and quickly absorbed; really cooling and soothing, and I felt it reduced my morning puffy eyes more quickly, and the dark circles' • 'didn't irritate my eyes, cause spots or affect my make-up: I would definitely buy this' • 'eye make-up went on better because

my lids were smoother; good pick-me-up and great that it can be used under or over make-up' • 'the light tapping action they suggest was very helpful'.

 Skinvitals Eye Brighten Cloth Eye Treatment Mask

 7/10 These half-moon-shaped pads are drenched in ingredients, including liquorice root extract, ginger root oil, vitamin C and lemon (alongside a lengthy list of synthetics). The invigorating elements are said to brighten tired eyes and target shadows in 15 minutes; then you wipe away any excess. Although they are inexpensive individually, we recommend these one-use sachets for a tired-eye SOS only, as, used regularly, they'd become more bank-account challenging.

Testers say: 'Colourful, quirky packaging, and great to keep in

we love

your car or office drawer; just in case you go out and need a bit of a pick-me-up! Eye area looked brightened and lifted, dark circles less obvious' • 'feels cool and relaxing on eye area; made it look smoother and refreshed; really reduced dark circles – by over 50 per cent: but do remove eye make-up first!' • 'ten out of ten: eyes felt lighter and looked brighter; definitely reduction in puffiness – I would buy again' • 'bit weird looking, but easy to do; fine lines seemed less prominent, dark circles definitely lighter'.

Garnier Nutritionist Caffeine Eye Roll-on

6.75/10 The caffeine-boosted formulation in this slim applicator is applied with a cooling metal 'rollerball', which helps massage away fluid in the eye zone while delivering its microcirculation-boosting ingredients. It incorporates caffeine and pro-vitamin B5.

Testers say: 'Eyes did feel a lot more refreshed – and tightened (almost too much); goes on quite easily before make-up, though still needed eye cream, or fine lines seemed to remain apparent' • 'product rolled on easily and eyes felt wonderful! Fresh and awake' • 'I really liked the cooling effect' • 'this worked the morning after a long night out! Went on very easily and dried ready for make-up' • 'eyes looked brighter and clearer, skin less dull and tired. Friends noticed I looked more revitalised: it now lives in the nappy bag'.

Organic Surge Pure Extracts Eye Gel

6.37/10 Organic Surge products are free from parabens, SLS, synthetic perfumes, petroleum and chemical antioxidants. Cooling ingredients refresh the eye, and it also delivers calming camomile, antioxidant green tea and put-the-sparkle-back eyebright.

Testers say: 'Very easy to dispense and apply; eyes felt perked up – nice base for eye make-up, which went on beautifully; the perfect foil to small, sleepless children, slight hangovers and too much time at the computer' • 'wrinkles round my eyes looked less defined; got rid of my morning eye wrinkle, which I call a "scar" – amazing'.

Champneys Super Cooling Eye Rescue Gel

6.33/10 Eye-soothing ingredients in this new entry include cucumber and butcher's broom (a botanical known for its power to reduce puffiness and dark circles). Champneys suggest enhancing the cooling action still further by keeping it in the fridge for real puffiness crises!

Testers say: 'I loved this teeny, tiny glass tub of gel which made my eyes look clearer and more awake, even on tired days; very good at reducing puffiness' • 'eyes felt refreshed, cooler and less tired; good on puffiness – you only need a little' • 'eyes looked as if I'd had a good night's sleep' • 'didn't interfere with make-up once it had sunk in – about five minutes' • 'does a good job of smoothing out the eye area'.

how to make
salon treatments last longer

Many women invest a considerable sum in salon hair cut and colour – and maybe a manicure and eyebrow shaping. So here are some practical tips on prolonging those valuable salon treatments

Keep your hair colour vibrant

The day before colouring (at home or in salon), wash with a clarifying shampoo to remove excess build-up of products, so the colour penetrates deeper and lasts longer.

After colouring, wait at least two – preferably three – days before shampooing, so the pigment is fully sealed in the hair shaft.

Harsh detergents fade hair, so use a gentle moisturising shampoo designed specifically for colour-treated hair, and rinse with tepid water: hot water expands the cuticle, degrading colour.

Don't get into the habit of shampooing daily. Every two or three days is

plenty – less, if you live in the country.

After three weeks or so, use a colour-depositing shampoo which leaves semi-permanent pigment in your hair. Do this weekly, not more, as it can change the professional colour. (We know – Sarah's highlights went orange.)

Use a conditioner and/or styling aid with built-in sunscreens to prevent the sun fading your shade.

And wear a hat! Choose one that's big brimmed and close woven: it will protect your face and eyes, too.

Colour glazes are the newest high-tech product for reviving hue and shine. John Frieda's Luminous Color Glaze is beloved by hair junkies and

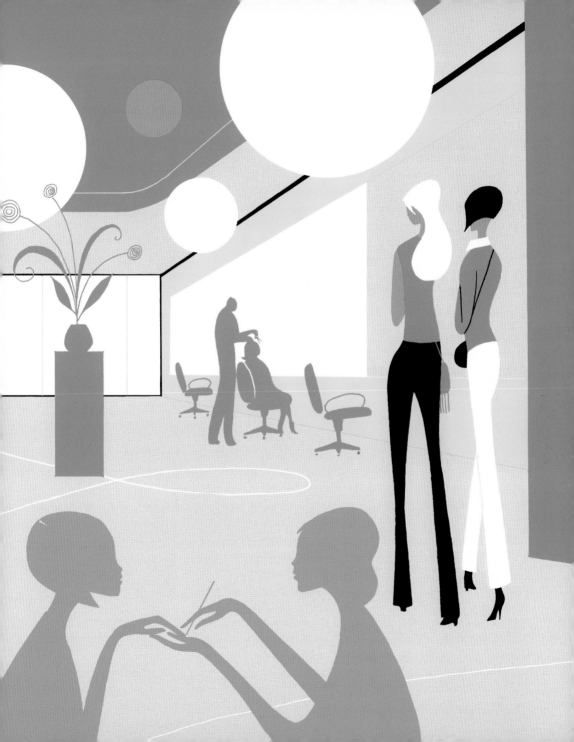

beauty editors – in three shades, plus Clear Shine.

Before using heated styling tools (drier, straightener, etc), spritz on a thermal protection spray such as Dove Heat Defense Therapy Mist, which contains polymers to prevent heat from getting into hair shafts and breaking down dye molecules.

Switch to an ionic blow-dryer with tourmaline (one of our favourite tips from Manhattan-based organic hairdresser John Masters); these are claimed to emit negative ions that seal the cuticle layer, giving smoother hair and keeping in colour.

Camouflage stray greys and roots with mascara: use an eyelash product or a specific hair version (budget brands include The Body Shop).

Prolong your hair cut

● Spend as much as you can afford.
● Choose an experienced stylist: the cut will almost always last longer than one from a novice.
● Consider growing your hair longer: it needs trimming less, though it may cost more in products.
● If you choose short hair, which often needs a monthly trim, go for a style that grows out well.
● After a cut, keep the ends hydrated with a daily leave-in conditioner, just on the ends.
● If ends or other bits look frizzy/fuzzy, smooth them with a titchy bit of oil, balm or Vaseline.
● Trim a fringe (bangs, to our American friends) with a pair of really sharp scissors on dry hair; the key is to hold them at a slant – never cut straight across – and snip a little bit, a lock at a time. You can't stick it back on, but you can trim a bit more.

DIY colour

If you colour your hair at home, stay within a couple of shades of your natural colour, otherwise the retouching is a big challenge – and nothing looks worse than half-grown-out colour. Whatever the shade, shun harsh tones: keep it soft and subtle, especially if you have pink cheeks. Also, avoid flat colour, which is unnatural and ageing: look for products that reflect the natural variations of colour in hair (L'Oréal has tone-on-tone and multi-tonal options).

Protect painted fingernails

This is a real case of do as we say, not as we do – since Sarah's fingernails, in particular, are the despair of manicurists. (It's down to horses, picking up flints in her field, and gardening – yes, she puts on gloves, but still the mud and wet get through.)

Ask for your cuticles to be pushed back, not cut – which makes them raggedy-looking faster. (We don't like our cuticles cut anyway.)

If you have weak nails, never let them be buffed in that full-on assault manicurists adopt to achieve a smooth surface. Your nails will be weak for months. A very gentle buffing once a month to keep bare nails rosy may help, but you will get a better effect by massaging them with nail oil daily.

Choose a light shade of polish for fingernails – it won't show chips as much.

Take your own polish to the salon, if possible, so you can do touch-ups at home.

After a manicure, apply a cuticle cream or oil to keep them supple, and paint on a clear topcoat to protect the polish. Do both of these daily.

Moisturise frequently – every time you wash your hands – and rub in oil whenever you can, particularly at night.

Wear gloves! Oh, and try digging your nails into a bar of soap (or a jar of balm or Vaseline) before you tackle tough-on-nails tasks, so the dirt floats out when you wash them.

'Choose a light shade of polish for fingernails — it won't show chips as much'

Keep brows in line

If you decide to invest in professional brow shaping, it will take about four weeks for the hairs to grow back (whether they are tweezed, waxed or threaded, it's all the same).

● Keep them tidy on a daily basis, using angled tweezers to pluck out any stray hairs between your brows or under the arch.

● Don't use a magnifying mirror, because it distorts the shape and you risk over-tweezing.

● For an expert look, fill in your brows with a matching pencil (see page 40), brush up and then out with an old, clean mascara brush, then set with brow gel, hair spray or a lick of balm.

tried & tested
facial scrubs

Just because you're going for a budget product to buff and scruff away those dull, dead skin cells, doesn't mean you'll settle for something scratchy and/or gummy on your precious face. These ticked our testers' boxes: effective, pleasant to use, complexion brightening – but rough? Certainly not. (NB: some very sensitive skins may not be suitable for scrubs– see 'we love' and 'tip', opposite.)

The Sanctuary Warming Microdermabrasion Polish

 7.75/10 This (like The Body Shop's winning facial mask, page 72) has a self-heating 'thermal action', when massaged into skin, with a gentle microbrasion (as they call it) action from natural earth and detoxifying kaolin. Jojoba, bamboo and beeswax make it skin softening as well, and The Sanctuary promise it will 'reduce the appearance of fine lines'. Here's the testers' verdict…

Testers say: 'Thick, creamy texture, with very fine gentle grains that heated with rubbing and stayed warm for a moment; skin felt soft and looked glowy after – really smooth, too' • 'the warmth felt very calming and luxurious; skin smoother, cleaner, lighter and brighter' • 'grain felt great, and skin more polished' • 'I test scrubs on my hands first – test hand was soothed and smoothed, paler, less prominent veins and pores, and less red'.

Organic Surge Pure Extracts Facial Exfoliant ❀

 7.66/10 With 'spirit-lifting' extracts of organic essential oils of rosemary and lemon, this is based on ultra-fine particles of apricot stone and walnut-shell particles together with nourishing almond oil and the soothing power of camomile and green tea. Organic Surge's range is free from parabens, SLS, synthetic perfume, mineral oils and skin-stripping foaming agents, but isn't quite as 'organic' as the name suggests. Some testers loved this; two others found it too poweful.

Testers say: 'Loved this luxurious nourishing cream, with its easy-flick lid tube. My 13-year-old daughter said, 'Mum, you are looking beautiful lately…your skin looks lovely and glowing' • 'grains were small and didn't scratch or irritate my skin, which is definitely brighter

and very soft'•'top marks
for their support for African
orphans'•'much more subtle
and suitable for regular use than
my usual scrub'.

Yes to Carrots C is for Clean Gentle Exfoliating Facial Cleanser ✿

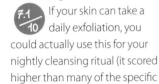 If your skin can take a
daily exfoliation, you
could actually use this for your
nightly cleansing ritual (it scored
higher than many of the specific
cleansers we trialled). Another
triumph for Yes to Carrots, this

we love

**Actually, we don't
go in for exfoliators
much at all – you can
count on one hand the
times either of us has
used them in the past
couple of years – but
that's because we
rely on the daily light
buffing action of a
muslin cloth (the type
you can buy from Liz
Earle Naturally Active,
or organic beauty
websites). One less
product to clutter the
bathroom shelf.**

one formulated with Dead Sea
mud, carrot juice and particles
of apricot. (We can't wait to put
their Yes to Tomatoes and Yes to
Cucumbers products through
their paces with our testers.)

Testers say: 'This is one of
the best scrubs I've used: very
gentle, not drying, pleasant to
use, easy to rinse off – and left
my sensitive skin smooth and
soft, especially helping with
dry flaky patches and
congestion'•'excellent economy
product; I would definitely
recommend it and buy it again'
•'my skin was glowing and
vibrant and felt soft; it has a
fine grain but gave a thorough
exfoliation'•'light, natural
fragrance and creamy texture'.

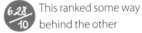 **Bioré Pore
Unclogging Scrub**

This ranked some way
behind the other
three 'steals' tested here, but we
felt it important to include as a
choice for oily/problem skins.
(In our experience, women with
troubled complexions are keen
consumers of scrubs.) It can
double as a daily cleanser, if you
wish: a creamy, pearlescent,
lightly foaming formula with
micro-beads and salicylic acid
to unclog pores and remove
dead skin.

tip

**If for any reason an
exfoliator irritates your
skin, try this tip from
New York dermatologist
Dr Patricia Wexler:
'Soak a washcloth in
equal parts ice-cold
skimmed milk and
cold water. Hold the
washcloth against your
face for five minutes.
This treatment is also
ideal for soothing
sunburns…' Or, indeed,
for any time your
skin is feeling touchy,
come to that.**

Testers say: 'Immediately, my
skin felt quite soft and looked
less grey; after a month, it looks
smoother and clearer. I was
very surprised – it's so creamy I
thought it would be useless, but
it's turned out to be really good
and gentle'•'hint-of-mint spa
smell, easy-squeezy tube and
product spread well over my
skin'•'very good product, with
soft grains, lovely smell – left
my skin clean and refreshed
with a subtle glow'.

tried & tested
face masks

A face mask can really transform your skin when it's got the blahs. The 'winner' in this category did better than dozens of chichi brands we trialled, and also the other masks featured here, which had a more mixed reception, albeit with some fervent fans.

The Body Shop Warming Mineral Mask

8.87/10 A truly stellar score for this 'self-heating' mask, which warms on contact with the skin, drawing out impurities (thanks to the kaolin and essential oils), while hydrating with seaweed extract. This five-minute rejuvenating skin blitz turns on the heat with a combination of ginger and cinnamon oils (plus a mineral called zeolite), and you'll also experience the antioxidant benefits of vitamin E.

Testers say: 'My skin is brighter and smoother; I liked the warming action and would definitely buy this in future' • 'my partner commented that my face looked "rested" after use' • 'skin looked cleaner, more radiant and shiny (in a good way!) – good value for money' • 'one of those rare, miracle products; skin clear, fresh and bright, and, most significantly, the rather large pores around my nose looked smaller – hooray!' • 'the warmth is like magic: you put it on, spread it around and it heats up and is superb – love it' • 'velvety-soft skin; I don't usually find time for face masks, but, having tried this, I'm converted' • 'a great mask before a night out – the rosy glow lasts a few hours; I suffer from dull skin and using this once a week really improved it. Who needs a face peel when you can buy this?'.

we love

As an exponent of home-made beauty treats, Jo tends to whiz up her own face masks with store-cupboard/fridge finds, a favourite being thick greek yogurt swirled with runny honey, which moisturises and brightens (that's the lactic acid). The only challenge is not eating it first.

Yes to Carrots C The Difference Exfoliating and Soothing Mud Mask

7.5/10 The combination of skin brighteners in this five-minute mask includes exfoliating jojoba beads, Dead Sea mud, carrot seed and avocado oils, carrot juice and

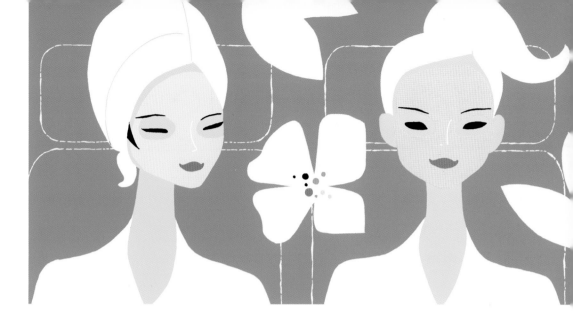

magnesium salts, along with high levels of antioxidants.

Testers say: 'Top marks! My skin was immediately even toned, smooth, glowing and felt very soft; such a pleasure to use – took five minutes and the results were excellent' • 'I can't praise this enough: it will be in my bathroom for ever!' • 'love the fact it's natural; my congested T-zone – which had blackheads – has cleared and my skin tone is much more even' • 'it's quality, economical, pleasant to use – what more could you ask for?' • 'the results are more noticeable than my much more expensive papaya peel' • 'easy to apply, lovely to use – by far one of the most effective masks I've used' • 'made me feel relaxed and revitalised, and my skin was brighter, tighter and plumper, with a luminous glow'.

 Skin Wisdom Daily Care Detox Thermal Mask (single use) This deep-cleansing warming treatment, created by Bharti Vyas, is based on rose clay and sweet almond oil, with green tea and soothing camomile. Skin Wisdom suggest damping the face before applying the mask.

Testers say: 'My skin looked refreshed, with a nice peachy glow, also tighter and firmer, and as if a lot of the oil had gone: it looked great the next day, very fresh and soft' • 'I will definitely be treating myself to one a week from now on, as the results were great, and it was nice to spoil myself and relax' • 'loved the nice warming effect and skin immediately felt fresh and awake, glowing, brighter and plumper' • 'make-up went on like a dream after using this' • 'skin looked glowing but not red; pores seemed minimised' • 'too much for one application for me, so I would probably use on "face mask night" with friends' • 'people said my face looked "amazing" after'.

tried & tested
facial oils

There are very few inexpensive facial oils on the market – perhaps because it's still considered that only 'sophisticated' skincare lovers get the nourishing, age-defying point of them. So most products here come in at over a tenner, but are still as much as £50 less than some other 'skin-vestment' oils in our other books and do last for ages. We suggest you consider making your own – see recipes opposite.

A'kin Rosehip Oil ❋ ❋ ❋

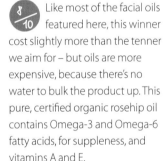

8/10 Like most of the facial oils featured here, this winner cost slightly more than the tenner we aim for – but oils are more expensive, because there's no water to bulk the product up. This pure, certified organic rosehip oil contains Omega-3 and Omega-6 fatty acids, for suppleness, and vitamins A and E.

Testers say: 'Skin felt velvety smooth and lovely instantly; no residue at all; makes my tired skin feel young and stretchy again' • 'my complexion looked really luminous, as if I had slept for a week; skin plumped, soft and younger; even my crow's feet not so noticeable' • 'fine lines finer and lip area smoother; small scar on my cheek much less noticeable'.

The Sanctuary Radiance Boosting Facial Oil ❋ ❋

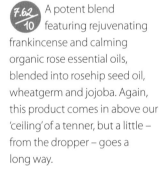

7.62/10 A potent blend featuring rejuvenating frankincense and calming organic rose essential oils, blended into rosehip seed oil, wheatgerm and jojoba. Again, this product comes in above our 'ceiling' of a tenner, but a little – from the dropper – goes a long way.

Testers say: 'Within 24 hours, my skin was soft and smooth; nice feeling – and bright' • 'skin smoother, well nourished, but not greasy or oily; my make-up went on really well next morning' • 'this product improved the texture of my skin' • 'after just three days, a colleague said my skin was glowing'.

The Body Shop Vitamin E Facial Oil

7.55/10 For normal and dry skins, The Body Shop recommends this oil as a 'pre-moisturiser treat'. It contains wheatgerm, rice bran and soya oils, all high in vitamin E, but is 'non-comedogenic' so it won't block pores. Most testers raved about it, but the 15ml bottle does bust our price 'ceiling'.

Testers say: 'I am a convert – my very dry face now looks and feels wonderful' • 'definitely enhances radiance – skin feels soft, plump and nourished; I use it night and morning and make-up goes on with no problem' • 'fine lines seem minimised' • 'loved the smell' • 'my skin felt softer and moisturised but a bit heavy for the eye area'.

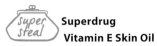 **Superdrug Vitamin E Skin Oil**

7.55/10 This tied with The Body Shop's entry. But we think it's a bit naughty to trumpet 'With naturally sourced vitamin E' on the front of your (30ml) bottle, in a product in which the first ingredient is mineral oil and the second is silicone, although it does also feature jojoba and olive oils. Still, this lightweight oil smells pretty and sinks in fast – and testers liked it.

Testers say: 'I was very impressed; the quality is as good as my expensive facial oil, and in some ways, it was better – less heavy and very easily absorbed; improved my acne-prone skin' • 'very cooling' • 'not a miracle cure but a simple and effective allrounder for a reasonable price' • 'I liked the almost almondy smell' • 'made my combination skin soft and moisturised, younger looking, better in texture and tone' • 'I'd recommend this to anyone thinking of trying a facial oil' • 'good for my very dry skin'.

Champneys Moisture Miracle Facial Oil ❀ ❀

6.88/10 Again, this is above our 'ceiling', but some testers went mad for it. Amazonian babassu oil and sweet almond

---

DIY facial oils

It's incredibly simple to make your own facial oils. You need a base oil (or blend of base oils), and some essential oils, which have different skin-enhancing properties. For each 30ml of base oil, add around 25 drops of essential oil in all. The least expensive way is to choose oils from the recipes below (you may already have some or all of them in your kit). We recommend Neal's Yard Remedies essential oils for their excellent quality.

Base oils for normal skin: jojoba, borage seed, evening primrose, carrot.

Add two or three of these: German camomile, geranium, lavender, rose, neroli, palmarosa, fennel, lemon.

Base oils for normal-to-oily skin: grapeseed, hazelnut, apricot kernel.

Add two or three of these: German camomile, juniper, geranium, lavender, cypress, palmarosa, lemon, rosemary, frankincense, marjoram.

Base oils for normal-to-dry skin: almond, jojoba, wheatgerm, olive oil, apricot kernel.

Add two or three of these: German camomile, calendula, lavender, sandalwood, patchouli, rose, calendula, geranium, neroli.

---

oil replenish the skin's lipid barrier, with vitamin E and a sense-pleasing essential oil blend including camomile, geranium and lavender.

Testers say: 'A wonderful product; my skin felt plumper, smoother, with loads more radiance – and such a tiny price, comparatively' • 'within 12 hours, my dry, flaky, mature skin looked plumped up and youthful! Excellent, easy to use and wonderful results!' • 'plumped up effect on skin; softening of lines round neck and corner of mouth' • 'gorgeous smell, and the oil alone got better results than my usual night cream' • 'great bottle with dropper, lovely product and a fraction of the price of my usual one' • 'best as a neck oil'.

 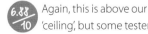

tried & tested
face 'fillers'

Fact: most of us are wusses, and, despite the Botox boom and fad for 'fillers', avoid the syringe. Hallelujah: the new trend is for 'faux fillers', aka 'line smoothers/blurrers', products you apply to your lines (under or over make-up) and – hey, presto! – they're gone. We've also given you the one (under-foundation) budget primer that did really well.

What's even more magic is that our trials revealed a couple of high-performers which cost much less than most. Although both of these do exceed our preferred £10 'ceiling', we feel they qualify as steals because a little goes such a l-o-n-g way. They also compare favourably with much pricier options: one upmarket rival product we trialled at the same time is priced at around £60, and scored far fewer points!

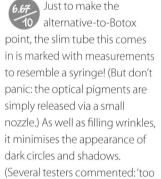

tip

Before these products were available, make-up artists used a pen-style concealer with light-reflecting pigments to stroke down lines (frown, nose-to-mouth, or mouth-to-chin lines). Patted in lightly, they blur wrinkles. Sarah does that, or uses a pale pink pencil by Valerie Beverly Hills as a filler.

L'Oréal Wrinkle De-Crease Collagen Filler Eye

6.67/10 Just to make the alternative-to-Botox point, the slim tube this comes in is marked with measurements to resemble a syringe! (But don't panic: the optical pigments are simply released via a small nozzle.) As well as filling wrinkles, it minimises the appearance of dark circles and shadows. (Several testers commented: 'too much packaging'.)

Testers say: 'Instant brightening of under-eye area; longer term it seems to be removing my dark circles'•'I now have two in my bathroom as standby'•'it really works; lines look immediately less obvious; general improvement of the skin around my eyes'•'a friend noticed improvement in line from my eyes to temples'•'easy to apply make-up after use; lines and crow's feet appeared diminished; fine lines were less noticeable'•'dotted around the eye contour, it made the area look brighter; I was impressed'.

L'Oréal Paris Wrinkle De-Crease Collagen Filler Double Action Lip & Lip Contour

6.5/10 As this name suggests, this is a lip multi-tasker: a dual-ended product which at one end dispenses anti-ageing 'collagen biospheres' (in L'Oreal-speak) and hyaluronic acid, a powerful moisturising molecule. The other end is more of a cosmetic 'filler', with the usual light-reflecting ingredients to create the immediate optical illusion of a smoother, less feathered lip line while you're waiting for the turn-back-the-clock ingredients to get to work. One of our testers reported that she knew it must be working because it tingled so much.

Testers say: 'Lipstick had a very good finish and looked "professional"; bit of a faff to apply but I've been pleased with the results' • 'simple, easy-to-use packaging; only needs a tiny amount of each cream; works well on the very fine lines around my top lip; lines are smoother and finer, and there is a definite improvement in the cupid's bow area, which looks much more defined and prominent after several weeks' use' • 'my husband commented that my lips looked fuller – lovely product, but took time to work' • 'didn't plump lips directly but definitely improved contour and made lip area more defined and smooth' • 'lips definitely appear plumper with that cream, which gave the impression of a lift'.

♡ we love

Of all the budget options she's tried, Jo would go for the **L'Oréal Wrinkle De-Crease Collagen Filler Eye** – but, to be honest, she's unswervingly devoted to a product called **Tri-Aktiline**. The cost is about double that of these, but so little is needed to fill lines ('especially the squint-related one between my brows') that she figures her tube will probably last her the rest of the century. In fact, it has become the most important product in her make-up kit.

Or try a make-up primer…
There are precious few affordable make-up primers around yet (although we predict a rush in the next couple of years). Make-up primers create a flawless canvas over which to apply foundation, concealer, etc, and help make-up last better. Again, these contain light-reflective and skin-smoothing particles. Of those trialled, the most inexpensive one that did well was by GOSH – slightly over a tenner, but read on.

GOSH Velvet Touch Foundation Primer

 A very high score for the Danish GOSH brand (exclusive to Superdrug, as we went to press). You can tell this is rich in super-smoothing silicones from the velvety feel. Like most primers, it should ensure that make-up not only looks smoother, but stays put for longer. Testers mostly raved about this – and it scored higher than dozens of others, including some famous 'make-up professional' ranges.

Testers say: 'I would definitely buy this thick gel; sank in quickly, leaving skin velvet smooth; great base for foundation; friend said my skin looked very good – my foundation lasted all day' • 'ten out of ten! Brilliantly easy to apply, on top of moisturiser – my skin felt perfect! Foundation glided on. Now I couldn't live without this' • 'amazing: I'd never used a primer before but this has converted me' • 'left a thin silk-like finish on the skin, giving it a healthy, soft glow' • 'particularly good with my powdery-finish foundation' • 'I had been using an expensive primer but this works equally well – the only difference is the price' • 'the husband came through on this one, commenting on how good my skin looks'.

foot files

Don't think us crazy, but if we were limited to just five essential beauty products, a foot file would be on the list – because without happy feet, we can't feel (and therefore look) fabulous. And our testers' feet are much happier, too, now they've tested the contenders to discover these accessibly-priced foot-buffers.

Revlon Pedi-Expert

 An extremely high score for an extremely scary-looking object, which is a new entry in this category. The ergonomically curved pink handle fits the hand nicely, while on the other side is a high-quality cheese-grater-esque file, which clearly – from what our testers say – does the job of buffing away even the hardest skin and calluses. Several testers gave it full marks. **Testers say:** 'Ten out of ten for this bright pink, very well-designed, compact pod, with flat file and "grater", plus nail clippers; file has really smooth action, which worked best on dry/hard skin on heels: I love this' • 'perfect for big or small hands. I used this on wet soapy feet in the bath: it barely even tickled, but the hard skin was gone! Would DEFINITELY buy this' • 'used this just once, then a foot cream – and my feet were reborn!' • 'this truly deserves ten out of ten; I've been showing off my soft feet to everyone. Well done, Revlon!' • 'I used the grater first on the build-up of hard skin on the balls of my feet and around my heels; once that was under control I just used the plane to keep on top of it' • 'perfectly designed – what a fantastic product'.

tip

Our überpedicurist friend Bastien Gonzalez says that hard skin on feet should be buffed very, very lightly – so don't go at it all guns blazing, but just gently whisk skin away from the surface with your foot file. (He says dry, but Sarah finds damp skin much easier with feet, over a towel for easy cleaning.) Otherwise, he warns, 'the layers of skin become compacted and actually harder, and more uncomfortable to walk on.'

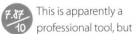

we love

No. We don't just love the Alida Foot File mentioned here, we love, love, love, love, love it, and have duly given it to all our friends – who then give it to all theirs, like some kind of gorgeous-foot chain letter. 'Nuff said?

Ms Pedicure 2 in 1 Callus Reducer

7.87/10 This is apparently a professional tool, but just brilliant for amateurs: it has a stainless-steel-surfaced file with a non-slip handle, and two sides – one for heavy-duty filing, the other for a final smooth down. (It's so effective that Ms Pedicure do caution: 'Use this reducer gently and regularly, but beware of over-smoothing your soles – feet like a nice bit of natural cushion to protect themselves.')

Testers say: 'Very easy to use; fits easily into hand; whisks away dry skin smoothly, not abrasively' • 'nice solid file that's easy to wash out; removed dry skin easily, without tearing or roughening skin' • 'my teenage daughter loved this, as it removed hard patches of skin on the sides of her toes and feet' • 'left feet smoother and softer, and, used gently, regularly, prevents build-up'.

Alida Tools That Assist Dual-Sided Foot File

7.14/10 With its green rubber ergonomically designed handle (making it a cinch to hold), this is like a gentler version of a Microplane cheese grater – and personally (although it came third with our testers), we think that nothing we have ever trialled as beauty editors comes close. One side is rougher, one smoother – as with most foot files – and it just squeaks in under the tenner. PS: it's dishwasher safe for washing.

Testers say: 'Top marks; beautifully designed for the job; I thought it wasn't doing anything but was amazed at the results: soft, smooth, perfect skin. Excellent; I love it' • 'easy to use; files away dead skin very smoothly; best used on dry feet' • 'my skin felt really smooth and perfectly prepped for a foot cream after using this; I would hate to lose this and would rush out immediately to replace it

if I did' • 'the handle fitted my hand perfectly – and the file really got rid of dry skin' • 'very gentle; would be hard to over-file the skin with this'.

Carnation Footcare Corn and Callus Foot File

6.75/10 The advantage of the top foot files in this category – including this entry from Carnation – is that, because they're made of metal, they can be easily rinsed, for hygiene. Again, an easy-grip handle to this.

Testers say: 'Very user-friendly design; comfortable to use, and the curve makes it easy to apply the file where needed; has a smooth, non-abrasive action; my hard skin is much improved and not building up – very useful' • 'the right size for filing all areas of my foot, and easy to wash after use' • 'effective, and I would definitely use it regularly, as my feet felt much better without the dead skin' • 'loved the effect this had on my feet; I was worried it would be harsh, but after use my feet felt much smoother and softer – great for getting feet into sandal-wearing condition'.

tried & tested
foot treats

Step one, you buff (see page 78 for the best foot files). Step two, you slather. Result? Happy feet. Our testers trialled dozens of affordably priced foot (and leg) revivers – and these not only had them skipping, but the scores outpaced many expensive rivals in this category.

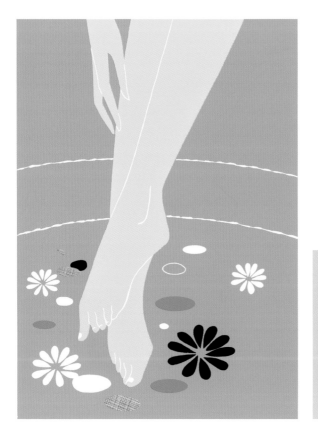

 Palmer's Cocoa Butter Leg Relief Massage Lotion

Menthol and lavender – which help relax swollen, achy muscles – give this rich lotion its cooling, refreshing action. It's designed mainly for legs, but our testers trialled it for feet, foremost. Shea butter, cocoa butter and vitamin E soften as it soothes.
Testers say: 'I really love this cream; so easy to use and quickly absorbed; really refreshed my feet and legs' • 'ten out of ten! Rich,

tip

To revive feet: fill a washing-up bowl with cool water, add five drops of peppermint essential oil, swish, and soak toes for ten minutes. (To combat hot-flush night sweats, try a foot wash in cold water before bed.)

luxurious, moisturising texture; fresh fragrance; skin felt beautiful – good after shaving' • 'relieved my swollen ankles' • 'good for tired muscles after running'.

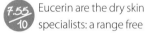

we love

It's been around for ever (since 1985, actually), but Jo has a nostalgic affection for the Body Shop's Polo-scented Peppermint Foot Lotion, *below,* also the Weleda Foot Balm, *left.* Sarah has to apply foot cream and/or balm religiously; her current 'squeeze' is Nivea SOS Relief Body Lotion for very dry skin, which works well and comes in a huge 200ml tube for almost a SuperSteal price.

Weleda Foot Balm ❀ ❀

8/10 Weleda grows its herbs biodynamically; this features antiseptic calendula, disinfectant and anti-fungal lavender, rosemary and myrrh, along with invigorating rosemary and zingy sweet orange. Weleda say it works as an antiperspirant deodorant for sweaty feet, too.
Testers say: 'I loved this – it absorbed really fast; no greasy residue' • 'made me feel as if I had new feet; reviving and refreshing' • 'loved the smell: uplifting, non-cloying' • 'my feet felt lighter'.

Eucerin Dry Skin Intensive Foot Cream

7.55/10 Eucerin are the dry skin specialists: a range free from perfume and colourants, clinically proven to boost moisture levels in the skin. This cream, is blended with glycerine, lipids, lactic acid and ten per cent urea to help reduce calluses and cracks. It's a whisker over our 'ceiling', but included for sensitive soles…
Testers say: 'Heaven! After a 15-hour day and two-hour flight,

this reduced the swelling on my hot, sticky feet' • 'very effective at softening the skin' • 'didn't have to use foot file as much, this worked so well' • 'left my feet like new'.

The Body Shop Peppermint Cooling Foot Lotion

7.14/10 A new entry for a really classic product: this truly minty pink lotion is a Body Shop 'hero', and has been reviving and softening Jo's feet (among many others!) for more decades than she dares to admit. Nowadays, the signature nourishing cocoa butter is Community Traded, from Ghana.
Testers say: 'Takes me back – in a good way – to being a teenager! One of the best foot lotions out there' • 'refreshing, soothing, lovely fresh smell – love it!' • 'rich enough to get rid of my dry skin; smell would kill any odours!' • 'improved my rough dry heels greatly' • 'used it when I was pregnant and it really relieved the water retention

in legs and feet, leaving them fresh and energised' • 'I spend all day on my feet at work and this made my feet more comfortable'.

Garnier Foot Cocoon

7.12/10 Combining lipids from olives, grapes, avocados, apricots and blackcurrants with softening glycerine, this is said to increase hydration by 69 per cent, an hour after application. It scooped several gongs before landing this Beauty Bible award.
Testers say: 'Reduced tiredness and soreness after a busy day shopping; pleasant, clean fragrance; legs felt refreshed, as if they'd been pampered by a professional: have bought more as gifts' • 'smelt summery and refreshed legs' • 'hydrated well' • 'I'm a sucker for anything that smells citrussy, so I liked this' • 'good value for money and does soften my feet; surprisingly non-greasy, after it had time to sink in'.

tried & tested
compact foundations

We can't claim that the scores for these inexpensive options knocked anyone's socks off as dramatically as the more luxurious brands, so we've only three to offer you – but they're still useful for beauty-hounds in search of a quick fix. They're a super-fast way to do your face, or for touch-ups (see tip, *opposite*). Some are creams which convert to powder; others start as a powder texture, and can be wetted for extra coverage. Do make sure you find the right shade for you (as always), and prep with a good moisturiser.

L'Oréal Infallible Make-up Long-Lasting Creamy Powder Foundation

 L'Oréal promise rather extravagantly that this 'resists make-up meltdown from morning until night' and most testers remarked on its dense coverage. The stay-put Infallible range includes a lipstick and liquid foundation as well as this handy compact powder-style base – which features a mirror and a sponge. Five shades are available: our testers were assigned 140 Beige Doré, a medium tone.

Testers say: 'Very portable and easy to apply with its own sponge; gave smooth, matt finish, which did even out skintone – looked natural; lasted as long as my usual base' • 'very easy, great coverage: covered blemishes; looked natural' • 'I found it difficult to apply with the little sponge it came with; putting it on with my fingers didn't work at all, but once I started using a proper foundation brush, it was a lot easier' • 'covered open pores quite well' • 'very natural looking, matt and smooth; covered some blemishes' • 'gave reasonably heavy coverage, but beware any dry patches – it really shows them up' • 'good budget product; definitely not mask-like but you need a good moisturiser first'.

The Body Shop All in One Face Base

 This one just squeaks in under our 'ceiling' – but the classy silver compact (which includes a separate compartment to accommodate the

Where compact foundations really score is for after-dark or desk-to-dinner face touch-ups. The texture of these products allows you to reapply easily later in the day, wherever needed. If you choose a powder formula, keep a small spray of rose water in your desk drawer and spritz the sponge to 'wet' it, before sweeping over your complexion to conceal flaws.

accompanying high-quality sponge, and an excellent mirror) justifies extra pennies. The formulation also includes antioxidant vitamin E as well as Community Trade marula oil (marula is a South African native tree, rich in skin-conditioning oleic acid), from a project which has helped more than 750 women and their families benefit from this harvest. There are five shades – these testers trialled 04, a mid-tone. Some liked it, but

others were unimpressed.

Testers say: 'Looks quite natural as long as you don't apply too much; matt effect, rather than dewy/glowing; looked better the less you apply; quite good on open pores' • 'a good alternative to liquid foundation: easy to apply and gives enough coverage to pop out to the shops; for someone with an even skintone it would be fine all the time' • 'one application was quite sheer; additional ones gave a much more "made-up" appearance; best applied with a damp sponge' • 'extremely easy to apply and stayed fixed to my face all day' • 'covered well; looked a bit powdery'.

Sleek MakeUP Oil-Free Crème to Powder Foundation

6/10 The perennial question we're asked is: which ranges offer great shades for darker complexions? So Asian and black readers will want to know about Sleek MakeUP – a really affordable (prices start at just 99p for eyeshadows!) alternative to brands such as Fashion Fair and Iman. There are shades to suit even the darkest skintones – although our testers tried the lightest, Bamboo 485, simply because it's easiest to match a

group of fairer-skinned testers than dark, who tend to have wider variations. Again, expect a full-size mirror and sponge in the black compact. Unlike the previous two entries, this concealing foundation starts as a soft, creamy, oil-free emulsion, then morphs into a matt, powder feel; it's available in a dozen shades that go as dark as Hot Chocolate and Deep Sable.

Testers say: 'At first it feels thick and oily but lighter on the skin, with a smooth texture; looked quite natural and seamless; gave good, even coverage' • 'stayed on well and covered blemishes, thread veins, etc' • 'very easy to apply smoothly with a foundation brush; great packaging; perfect to pop in your handbag and apply ad hoc, as required' • 'my skin looked very velvety and felt incredibly soft; covered thread veins, but it did settle in fine lines' • 'very comfortable; felt breathable and light, but not for mature or problem skins' • 'light, but quite matt, although it did not make skin look heavily made up; didn't go powdery or flaky; excellent to take out with you; works well to touch up liquid foundation, or on its own to even skintone – though you might need a concealer as well for blemishes'.

tried & tested
liquid
foundation

A foundation that doesn't match your skintone is no steal. So our advice with these face bases – which, despite the relatively low scores, our testers liked much more than those from several of the big brands – is to find the shade that blends seamlessly into your natural skintone (tested in daylight on your jawline) or look elsewhere...

Rimmel Lasting Finish 16 Hr Mineral-Enriched Foundation

6.94/10 With 'minerals' being the foundation buzzword, everyone seems to be jumping on the bandwagon. (In fact, most foundations have always been based on minerals.) Still, this product played well with our testers, who trialled the palest shade, 100 Ivory. Silicones and 'water-friendly polymers' give it its '16-hour transfer-resistance' (don't you love beautyspeak?), and the bevy of minerals all have known skin benefits.
Testers say: 'Really impressed – a great recession-busting product; almost matte finish but not powdery or cakey at all feels light, looks fresh and moisturising – covers better than my usual base' • 'long-lasting

> ## tip
>
> **If you feel your base is a bit heavy, mix it with a spot of moisturiser or primer first, in your palm, for a dewier, lighter look.**

formula really works; my make-up stayed in place all day – which never happens normally' • 'top marks: ideal consistency, very easy to apply with a sponge, blended and covered perfectly. Not too sheer or too thick' • 'quite sheer, but you can build up, for more coverage' • 'like the squeezy tube, so no gunk build-up!'.

Max Factor Miracle Touch Liquid Illusion Foundation

6.75/10 Make-up artist Pat McGrath worked on the development of this foundation, which melts into the skin as it warms, releasing pigments evenly, and then 'sets' to a powder finish. Although it comes in a compact, it's not really a compact foundation – more like a gel, according to one tester, which is why it's in this category. Our Beauty Bible babes trialled Creamy Ivory: some liked it a lot, some didn't. (NB: this just nudges in at over a tenner, but is still a steal when you compare it to the premium brands.)

Testers say: 'This was perfect for me, as I often do my make-up on the go; easy to apply with the sponge and blend in – so easy, I can do it without a mirror!' • 'very pleased with this; just as good as my usual foundation – and I didn't need my usual concealer' • 'this gave too much coverage for an everyday "natural" look for me, but good

tip

The problem with buying 'drugstore' brands like these is that testers aren't always available – and shade is soooo important. Shop at larger pharmacies, and you're more likely to find testers. If you're unsure, go lighter rather than darker.

for a night out' • 'evened out skin tone, covered small thread veins; didn't highlight pores, as some foundations do' • 'a bit messy for portable touch-ups' • 'liked the ease of use' • 'looked thicker than it was on the skin, which it left with a slightly dewy powder finish – very "finished"! – liked it, though touch-ups were tricky'.

e.l.f. Shielding Hydro Tint SPF15

6.55/10

What can you say about a foundation that costs less than a fiver but out-scores brands priced seven times as much? You may not get sexy packaging with e.l.f., but the contents of the slim, nozzled clear tube impressed our testers. This is a sort of hybrid tinted moisturiser/sheer foundation, with a pretty good SPF, too (but remember, it won't last all day). It comes in four 'tones' – our lot tried Tone 2.

Testers say: 'Excellent for everyday, and, combined with a concealer, for going out' • 'perfect for those who like a very natural look: evens out colour, gives a great base for blush/bronzer, and is so light as to be almost undetectable' • 'gives a dewy, soft, attractive sheen – very natural, but not if you're looking for a more groomed and finished feel' • 'left lovely healthy glow on cheeks; T-zone needed a bit of powder; covered most small blemishes' • 'initially I turned my nose up at this, but after some use, I far preferred it to my normal, expensive foundation!'.

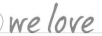

we love

Jo swears by Maybelline Pure Liquid Mineral Foundation: dewy, lightweight, blends well, but offers good coverage for broken veins, especially if used with a foundation brush.

more flash than cash

everyday summer

This soft glowing effect should suit most colourings.

The kit: liquid foundation, bronzing powder, eyeliner, mascara, lip gloss.

Make-up artist Jenny Jordan, who has beautified a galaxy of star faces, maintains you can spend much less, yet still look fab by choosing expensive-looking shades in cheap ranges. The prices are unbelievably low, all under a tenner and some SuperSteals under a fiver, making the 'cost per wear' teeny.

 MeMeMe Radiant Minerals Illuminating Foundation
Shade: six good options.
Jenny says: 'This liquid base is sheer, light, easy and quick to blend; let it sink in before applying bronzing powder. The design is great, and one pump per wear is plenty'.

Bourjois Mineral Radiance Pressed Powder
Shade: 07 Hâlé.
Jenny says: 'Use a large powder brush to whisk this soft-looking, matt-with-a-glow bronzing powder sparingly across cheeks, and other bits where you would get naturally tanned. This natural-looking bronzer also has teeny twinkles of gold, which is very flattering'.

 Rimmel Eyeliner Pencil
Shade: Brown.
Jenny says: 'Apply close to lashline; start top line above the outside of your eyeball, winging out, then smudge with a dry cotton bud for a velvety edge. I prefer brown eyeliner – black can make you look flat and tired. This dark rich coffee bean colour looks really good next to your eye, and enhances the white. A goldy, bronzey brown is lovely too, like M.A.C Teddy Eye Kohl'.

Max Factor Masterpiece Mascara
Shade: Brown/Black for day; Black for evening.

Jenny says: 'This is the best mascara yet, with creamy rich colour and a fab brush that glides through lashes, making them longer and longer. I've used it for over three years and nine out of ten clients say it's the best'.

 Collection 2000 Love Your Lips SPF20 Balmgloss
Shade: choose from pale-honey Tender, deeper-gold Delight, or rosy Adore.
Jenny says: 'This moisturising lip gloss, with a good sun screen, can vie with Chanel! It's comfortably unsticky, with rosehip and mango extracts to soothe and hydrate.'

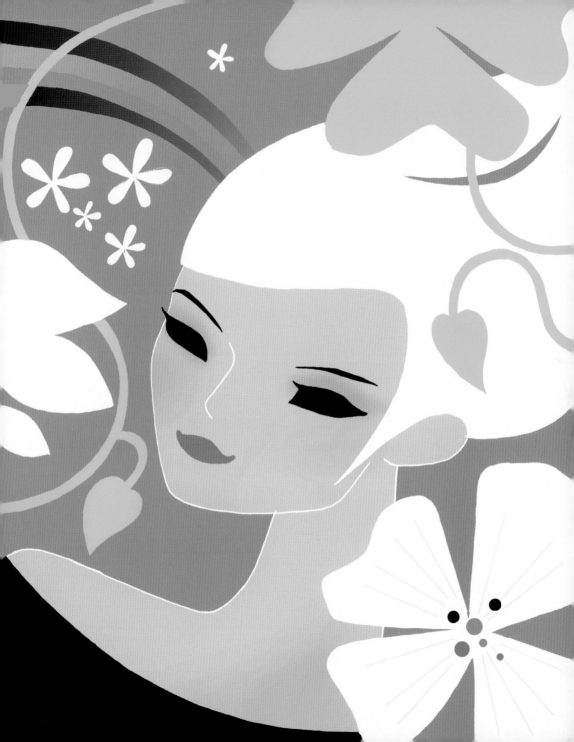

natural but better

With a little more coverage for those who need it, this collection still gives you a natural look for day.

The kit: foundation (optional), concealer, eyeshadow, mascara, eyelash curler, blush, lip gloss.

MeMeMe Radiant Minerals Illuminating Foundation (as in 'everyday summer', if wished).

Bourjois Imperfection Concealer
Shade: choose from three shades (coloured skins, see page 52).
Jenny says: 'Cheap concealers can be very drying, but this cute-looking creamy stick gives plenty of coverage and is spreadable enough for dark under-eye circles: do use over an eye cream around eyes, to avoid any crepiness showing through. Build up in very thin layers, tapping lightly into the skin with your ring finger. Also use on your eyelids as base, then powder lightly and apply eyeshadow.'

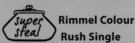 **Rimmel Colour Rush Single Eye Shadow**
Shade: Taupe.
Jenny says: 'Taupe is a really versatile colour and very flattering for everyone. It's never OTT, so you can rush it on in the morning. You can use this real multi-tasker on your brows, eyelids, and as an eyeliner. Brush it through your brows for definition, stroke on lids and/or in socket with a blender brush, then use it damp with a tiny paint brush to trace along your lash lines.'

Max Factor Masterpiece Mascara, as in 'everyday summer'.

 Rimmel 3 in 1 Powder Blush
Shade: Autumn Catwalk 003.
Jenny says: 'You can't go wrong with this palette, which gives you a light pink at one end, peach the other, with a sparkly rose in between – the perfect mix for a fresh but subtle effect. Sweep your blush brush five times over the whole surface, then knock off excess. Swirl from cheeks to temples, with a touch on earlobes. You could use the warmer colour on eyelids.'

Bourjois 3D Effect Lip Gloss
Shade: Rose Symbolic No 42.
Jenny says: 'This suits-all, rosy praline gloss glides on like a luxury brand and fades with subtle softness. For daytime, choose lippy colours a tone darker than your natural lips.'

day into evening

If you're going out straight from work and don't have the time or opportunity to take your make-up off and start again, freshen up by spritzing over your face and neck with mineral water, or make up your own complexion cocktail with filtered water and a few drops of rose water and glycerine. Then redo your skin (not forgetting base or concealer and powder on your eyelids and under – and right up to – your lower lash line). Then you can glam up eyes and lips with stronger colours – but don't go for broke with both: remember that you still need a bit of subtlety. Finally, set with a dusting of translucent powder (see page 156 for our testers' choices).

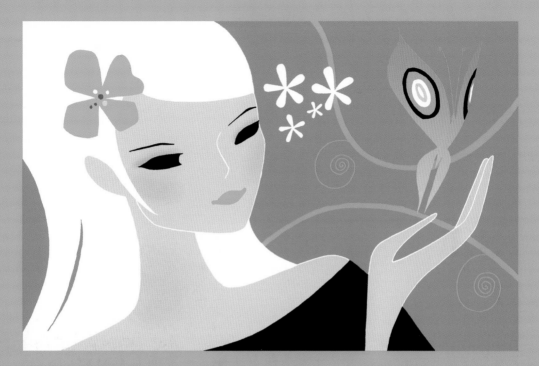

Skin: redo foundation and concealer where needed; sweep on bronzer and finish with translucent powder.

Eyes: try a coloured eyeliner pencil underneath your eyes (on top looks a bit dated). Navy blue looks fabulous on blondes, redheads and greys, as it flatters pale skins. Greens and blues – aquamarine/bottle/teal – are amazing on darker colourings. (Superdrug have a sensational range at amazing prices.)
If you have a darkish eyeshadow with a bit of sparkle, sweep some over your lids, then wet a fine brush and use it as eyeliner. We're mad about Bourjois Ombre Stretch in Brun Nylon, a slightly glimmering taupe that's worthy of Chanel.
Add a dab of highlighter under your browbone and on your cheekbone – also on your collarbone and between your breasts if they're on show.

Lips: gloss gives lips volume and oomph! Slick on a rich dark lip gloss (raspberry or plum shades look glam, especially for women of colour: Rimmel Vinyl 1000 Carat in Razzle Dazzle could get you noticed) or put lots of clear or natural lip gloss on top of your favourite lipstick.

Shimmer: spread a shimmer cream or powder across your cheekbones to the temples, on eyelids and over shoulders and décolleté to lift skin and give it lustre. (Nivea Visage Natural Beauty Radiance Boosting Moisturiser contains a subtle 'shimmer-iser' too).

tried & tested

hair masks

The fast-track to hair gorgeousness, these. And absolutely no reason to break the bank for them, as our testers' shining comments (and excellent scores) prove. So, just slather on once a week, as all top hairdressers prescribe, like good Beauty Bible babes…

Louise Galvin Natural Locks Deep Conditioning Treatment ❀

8.25/10 This appears in *The Green Beauty Bible*, but is also a 'steal' (just!), from A-list colourist Louise's more affordable 'diffusion' line. With no chemical 'nasties', it just contains lashings of good stuff for hair, including grapeseed oil, vegetable glycerine, jojoba, soy protein – infused with uplifting citrussy essential oils.

Testers say: 'I really liked this conditioner; easy to apply, lovely fragrance, made hair shiny and healthy-looking; but do follow the direction for double rinsing' • 'thick, creamy consistency which was really easy to work through hair; made hair smell fresh and clean' • 'managed frizz, and loads of people comment on the shine and bounce; very effective at enhancing the different tones in my hair'.

John Frieda Collection Frizz-Ease Miraculous Recovery

8/10 Described as a 'strengthening crème-masque', from the ground-breaking Frizz-Ease range, this is good for frizzy and curly hair, and dry hair, too – indeed, anyone looking for gloss, shine and enhanced 'resilience', as the anti-breakage formula is said to provide 'targeted conditioning to damaged areas'.

Testers say: 'Brilliant: my hair was really glossy and shiny straight after, and really soft – ten out of ten' • 'easy to apply, hair softer, glossier and more manageable' • 'let my hair fall and stay in style better' • 'excellent de-frizz factor; hair silky, manageable, and shiny'.

A'kin Intensive Moisture Vitamin Masque ❀

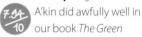

7.94/10 A'kin did awfully well in our book *The Green Beauty Bible*, but their products don't often qualify as 'steals'. This does: a mask targeted at dry or chemically treated hair (but which can be used on all hair types), with lots of active ingredients, including white tea, ginkgo and jojoba oil.

Testers say: 'Very easy to apply from squeezy tube; love the fresh smell; hair looked healthier and more glossy and was easier to blow-dry after' • 'my hair frizzes very easily but didn't do so, despite the damp weather' • 'love

this product: really did improve my hair's condition' • 'massive improvement; my mad, crazy, bushy hair looked…wonderful!'

 Andrew Collinge 1 Minute Wonder Deep Conditioning Treatment

7.71/10 With most hair masks, the longer you leave it on, the better – but this is for the I-want-it-now crowd: from highly respected Manchester-based UK hair 'name' Andrew Collinge, this takes just 60 seconds to deliver a powerful moisturising boost. Three testers scored it at ten.

Testers say: 'Top marks: very easily absorbed, hair was de-tangled, good sheen, soft and silky, didn't feel heavy – a bargain; haven't got the same results with

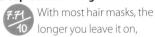

Jo actually nagged John Frieda about creating a hair mask for blonde hair, so he did (and got her to try the prototype) – and she's been loving Sheer Blonde Hair Repair ever since, to keep her highlights super-glossy.

higher-end products' • 'great condition and lovely loose curls; no frizz; like the "no parabens"; bad hair days can be banished!' • 'felt this was repairing my hair and the colour looks refreshed; now part of my beauty routine'.

 Organic Surge Citrus Mint Intensive Treatment ❀

7.71/10 The clue to the zesty, mood-boosting fragrance which so appealed to our testers is in the name of this product, which features organic lemon oil. (Organic Surge boast that their range is 'developed with no nasties or obscure chemicals for your precious skin to absorb'.)

Testers say: 'Hair was very soft and shiny, easier to comb through; frizz reduced' • 'minty, fresh smell' • 'fairly thick but easy to use on my long, thick hair; left a nice shine and my very dry ends looked healthy' • 'a small miracle the first time I used it – hair soft, shiny and healthy-looking' • 'the best hair mask I've tried'.

 1 Minute Wonder L'Oréal Elvive Re-Nutrition Replenishing Mask

7.33/10 Enriched with royal jelly, this infuses hair with

moisture in just one to two minutes, before rinsing, helping to boost manageability and bounce. (Clever L'Oréal advertise this with Penélope Cruz, as swingy-haired a beauty as we can think of.)

Testers say: 'Of all the products from Beauty Bible this was the most credit-crunch-tastic! My boyfriend said my hair swished like a shampoo ad, and loved the smell' • 'very easy to apply' • 'nice fragrance, like sweet honey'.

tried & tested
shampoo

There are loads of cheap shampoos. Oceans of them passed through our 'beauty dungeon' in Jo's house en route to our testers. It might not seem that something you wash out can make such a difference to how hair looks and feels – but as our testers found, a great shampoo does just that.

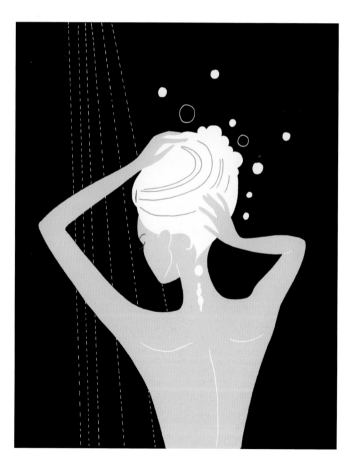

Louise Galvin Natural Locks Nourishing Shampoo for Dry/Damaged Hair ❋

8.28/10 The highest-scoring shampoo we've ever trialled is also a 'green' choice. The Galvins (offspring of Daniel Galvin, who was the late Princess of Wales's hair colourist) make a formidable hairdressing dynasty, with talented second-generation colourist Louise beating her brother Daniel into second place in this shampoo 'steal' category. The Natural Locks range is a 'sister' to Louise's pricy, 'cult' Sacred Locks range – and performs brilliantly, according to our testers, who awarded it a stellar score. It offers high levels of therapeutic natural ingredients – here, in this shampoo, targeted at thirsty hair, find provitamin B5, sweet almond extract and vegetable proteins, alongside gentle cleansers.

we love

Testers say: 'Ten out of ten! My hair was much more manageable and it transformed hair washing from a misery to a pleasure, as my hair knots so easily' • 'tricky at first, because it's quite runny; once I got the hang of it, was fine: lathered well on the second wash; easy to rinse out; left hair squeaky clean, shiny, bouncy, silky and light. I was very pleased' • 'no irritation to my occasionally itchy scalp' • 'great results – though needed conditioner too' • 'smells lovely – reminds me of a Chocolate Orange'.

Daniel Galvin Junior Hair Clinic Organic Hair Juice ❀ **8.06/10**

Daniel Galvin Jnr hails from a hairdressing dynasty, but he has rebelled against the 'conventional' haircare market, creating more natural products. This is one of two winners in this category formulated by Daniel: it's based on sodium cocosulfate (an ingredient not a million miles from sodium lauryl sulfate, we should point out, but less refined – and less irritating). Accessibly priced, this comes in two versions: Honeydew Melon, which our testers trialled, and Ginger & Lime.

We've both long been devoted clients at John Frieda's salons, where the product used on Jo's hair for a weekly blow-dry (which stays perfectly in place until her next visit) is John Frieda Sheer Blonde Colour Renew Shampoo. She loves the lavender fragrance and super-glossing effect (the UV filters are useful, too, for when she's on the beach).

Testers say: 'I normally dread washing my long hair because it takes such a long time, but I really enjoyed this, partly because of the wonderful honeydew melon fragrance; it left my hair beautifully clean, and gave it more volume and bounce – full marks!' • 'very effective product; left my hair squeaky clean, with no hint of residue, nicely shiny and smooth; easy to put a comb through, too' • 'loved this shampoo! Smell and texture were great; really practical packaging; my hair looked really shiny and healthy – fantastic product: can't find any complaints'.

John Frieda Sheer Blonde Tone-Refreshing Shampoo

7.87/10 John Frieda pioneered the idea of targeting different hair colours with specific products to bring out the natural beauty of that tone, and deal with any particular challenges. In this case, the shampoo is designed to neutralise brassy tones, using optical brighteners for brighter hair in just three washes.

Testers say: 'Very practical packaging; foamed well, giving a lovely rich dense lather; hair felt very clean and invigorated; easy to rinse out; no stinging; my hair looked very glossy; blonde highlights definitely enhanced; was manageable and soft' • 'I like almost everything about this product, and, despite the chemicals, would buy it, as I am won over by the results' • 'helped keep my colour true, had a lovely texture and performed well; would definitely buy' • 'hair glossy, brighter and definitely silkier' • 'liked the lavender smell; made my highlights sparkle and took out any old dulling – would definitely use this' • 'brightened my blonde hair and got rid of brassy yellow tones; hair felt lighter and more manageable'.

Tommyguns Fig, Plum & Marshmallow Shampoo

 7.62/10 Specifically for 'frizzy, chaotic and unruly' hairtypes, this has smoothing and softening fig, enriching plum, and marshmallow to boost hair elasticity.

Testers say: 'Smelt natural and appealing, subtly feminine; did a good job at cleaning; no stinging eyes, which was nice' • 'worked as well as anything I've ever tried, with the bonus that it didn't smell like air-freshener, as some cheap shampoos do' • 'lathered very well, and I was really happy with the results; hair was soft and easy to manage; also helps with "the frizz", as it says' • 'I just want a shampoo (and conditioner) that gives my hair a sleek, no-frizz look, and this delivered' • 'lovely figgy smell: my favourite thing about the product' • 'good results with my daily wash, especially when used with its complementary conditioner'.

John Frieda Brilliant Brunette Lustrous Touch Smoothing Shampoo

7.44/10 Although the Brilliant Brunette is supposedly targeted at – yes, brunettes – we sent it to testers with various hair colours, because we know that the 'satin finisher' ingredients (including jojoba oil, coconut oil and silk amino acids) can work their magic on pretty much anyone's bonce.

Testers say: 'Very glossy; enhanced colour; soft and manageable hair, but not too limp; my hairdresser noticed the colour difference and was very impressed!' • 'gave my blonde hair a soft, natural gloss and didn't darken it at all: I enjoyed using it' • 'liked the easy flip-top lid and the slight perfume' • 'felt and looked expensive; a little product goes a long way; my hair felt fresh and light after using it, but it always needed a conditioner' • 'fantastic: gives really smooth, shiny hair, and shimmering highlights – felt lovely and light but not flyaway – and didn't need any conditioner'.

Lee Stafford Climate Control Shampoo

7.33/10 This is the shampoo that goes with the conditioner which did well in our Tried & Tested on page 96, formulated to combat the challenges of frizz, particularly when it's weather related, and based on what they rather romantically call a Liquid Umbrella Technology™. Some mixed reviews (it gave one tester an itchy scalp), but if it suited testers' mops, they really loved it.

Testers say: 'Very smooth and easy to work into hair; felt it cleaned hair very well, and it seemed slightly glossier' • 'nice light perfume; gave me the most fantastic shiny hair; soft, minimal frizz, even without using conditioner – which I tried as an experiment; looked great when I let it dry naturally' • 'quite lubricating and de-tangling, but I always have to use conditioner too, on my thick curls' • 'only problem was that it contains SLS/SLES' • 'smelt a bit like bubblegum, but appealing – helped tame my frizz, over time'.

Save money – and scalp irritation – by skipping a second shampoo. Unless you've been doing something filthy (like cleaning out a cobwebby attic, paintballing – or wearing a riding helmet nearly daily, in Sarah's case), there's really no need. If the first shampoo doesn't froth adequately, add a bit more water.

tried & tested
conditioner

Most of us are searching for a not-too-heavy rinse to help detangle hair after shampooing. Well, heaven knows, there are lots out there: our testers combed (literally) their way through 40-plus entries in this category, which threw up some very good scores.

So there's definitely no need to pay over a hundred quid – yes, £100 – for a conditioner, which is the incredible price tag on one upmarket hair product out there. It does deliver pretty fab results (we've tried it) – but we'd rather have a night in a B&B with dinner, thanks, for that price!

Daniel Galvin Junior Hair Clinic Hangover Hair Organic Lavender Conditioner ❋

8/10 This has already featured in our book *The Green Beauty Bible* – but despite being sent vats of conditioners for this particular volume, we found that none of them did better, so here it is again. (If something's good, it's good! End of story.) Designed to 'detox and revitalise' even the most stressed-out tresses, it also comes in a Lemongrass & Lime option. (Although the name suggests it's organic, that claim's not certified by an organic body.)

Testers say: 'Good basic detangler and excellent for the price' • 'hair was more manageable and easier to comb through' • 'I stayed in steamy shower and bathroom for 20 minutes and it worked well' • 'pleasant lavender fragrance and practical packaging' • 'impressive gloss and good defrizz factor; brought my naturally curly, grey hair to fuller, shinier life – my husband commented on how nice it looked'.

John Frieda Weather Works by Frizz-Ease™ Daily Conditioner

 We're actually chuffed to bits that John Frieda has two top-ranking conditioners – because, for years, we've been going to his salons to have our hair done, and are pleased that our testers recognise that the products their stylists use in-salon – also widely available on every high street – really are top notch. This product is ideal for hair that tends to frizz in rain and sultry weather, with a special 'shielding technology' for humidity resistance, static control and UV protection.
Testers say: 'Really gorgeous fragrance; how fresh hair should smell – very easy to work through hair, and gave me lovely soft, shiny hair, which is much less flyaway and static, with no frizz at all, and didn't weigh it down' • 'little went a long way; gave a nice gloss' • 'despite cold wet weather, which usually makes my hair really static, dull and frizzy, there was hardly any with this – very

impressive!' • 'I used too much at first; when I used less, it was good for my dry, coarse and coloured hair; excellent, and I will definitely buy'.

 ### Herbal Essences Hello Hydration Moisture & Shine Conditioner

 Targeted at dry and damaged hair, this is quite highly fragranced – but we rather love the exotic scent, actually (imagine jasmine and coconuts, rather than orchid). Herbal Essences say it takes you on a 'multi-sensorial experience', being formulated like a fine fragrance, rather than a shampoo. (Oh, and our testers also liked what it did for their hair, not just their noses.)
Testers say: 'This product is excellent: beats other more expensive brands; left my hair

tip

If you want a 'kitchen' steal, try a cup of apple cider vinegar. (Trust us: it works – and not just on hair; it's a great fabric conditioner, too!)

shiny and manageable and less prone to frizz, even when I got caught in a shower' • 'I wash my hair daily, usually without a conditioner, but this was nice and left it better conditioned and a bit shinier' • 'excellent and great value for money; I have a really dry scalp and this is one of the few conditioners that doesn't irritate it and doesn't dry it out' • 'my hair was easier to comb through – shiny, but not heavy – and my highlights didn't look like straw!'.

Lee Stafford Climate Control Conditioner

This is part of Lee Stafford's 'three-step regime' for frizzy hair, but we trialled all the steps separately. Amazingly and impressively, out of the dozens of products that we tried in each category – shampoo, conditioner and frizz-tamers – all three did well enough to be included in this book (which augurs well for the synergistic benefits, when the products are used together). This sets out to 'weatherproof' hair, with UV protectors, and moisture regulators to help fight flyaway and unruly hair.
Testers say: 'I did notice a difference, particularly on the

second day, because my hair seemed to keep its style better; when I straightened my hair, it still looked good the day after' • 'good product if you use conditioner regularly' • 'lovely light, airy fragrance; I noticed a real difference in my coloured hair, which can be dry and frizzy, but instead looked shiny and healthy, smooth and silky – and was easier to style' • 'I liked this conditioner because it did what it said on the label'.

John Frieda Luxurious Volume Thickening Conditioner

 For hair that needs extra va-va-voom, this fortifies fine hair, without weighing it down. John Frieda tell us that it reduces static (a particular challenge with fine hair), to prevent flyaways, while enhancing hair elasticity and boosting shine and gloss.

Testers say: 'I've never been inspired by a hair product before but now I want to go out and buy the whole range! Gave lots of body and good gloss; made my dyed blonde hair look healthy; kept volume and shine for up to three days' • 'hair felt soft and light, and less fine and flyaway' • 'ten out of ten! Very

we love

♡

pleasant, appley fragrance; worked through hair easily; got a better shine than most other conditioners I've tried; hair appeared and felt thicker, so I quite often washed and left it, rather than having to blow-dry' • 'I am really impressed with this: a great discovery! A bit more than I usually spend, but worth it for my thinnish, flattish hair – and no itchy scalp'.

Dr. Organic 100% Organic Pomegranate Conditioner ✿

 From a Holland & Barrett range which has hugely impressed us, this lightweight conditioner is packed with antioxidants (pomegranate's signature compounds), so it's said to 'protect against the damaging effects of environmental stresses'. Conditioning and revitalising elements include

aloe vera, shea butter, milk protein, panthenol and sunflower oil, and it has a sense-enlivening tangy scent – prettily pomegranate-y, we would say.

Testers say: 'Not too thick, so spreads well; hair combed through easily after, with no tangles; reasonable frizz control' • 'pleasant, fruity smell – quite edible! Delivered a fantastic shine; hair felt soft and swish; would be great for normal hair, but not up to dry and coarse' • 'very easy, light texture and distributed easily through hair; easy to comb through, with no tugs or knots' • 'hair looked glossy and shiny, felt nourished and soft, without making it unmanageable or flyaway; didn't weigh hair down or make it greasy' • 'good product, left my hair feeling nourished and well conditioned; good effects'.

tried & tested
frizz-tamers

'The frizzies' turn women into desperate creatures. We have friends who scuttle into doorways at the merest hint of drizzle, and carry silk scarves in their bag to shield hair from rain. So defrizzing products can be literally life transforming – and, even better news: they're almost all 'steals'.

Toni & Guy Tame-It Serum

 A lightweight, pump-action serum from Toni & Guy's colour-coded 'Style ID' system (pink = for curls). The pros at Toni & Guy promise 'untameable, wayward hair with a tendency towards frizz' will surrender, acquiring a high-shine, flawless finish. An impressive score – though one tester complained of 'too much shine'.

Testers say: 'Very easy to smooth into my curly, dry, prone-to-frizz hair; gave an even coating with little effort, though I had to use three times the specified amount (as usual); hair was less frizzy, more manageable, smoother, curls defined' • 'invisible and unfeelable in hair – surprisingly effective' • 'very good at defrizzing my fine, thick, wiry hair' • 'passed the ultimate test: digging my veg patch on a sunny, windy day: it fared well – I didn't end up looking like Medusa!'

Lee Stafford Climate Control Protection Spray

 We should probably crown Lee Stafford the 'King of the Flyaways': his frizz-busting range has done supremely well in our T&Ts. The key is, apparently, Liquid Umbrella Technology™, which shields the hair cuticle. This is more akin to a hairspray than a serum, to help weatherproof hair that goes haywire in hot, wet and windy climates.

Testers say: 'Good defrizzer; very pleasing, healthy shine; hair looked lovely – and it survived a day gardening in the Shropshire wind' • 'my daughter-in-law tried to make off with this' • 'my hair needed far less use of the straightening irons – but don't use too much' • 'wind and weather is death to my hair, but this helped keep it well tamed'.

Samy Silk The Ultimate Anti-Frizz Smoothing Serum

 This ultra-lightweight mist is said to be as effective at controlling frizz as a liquid serum, but less messy to use. It can be sprayed on to wet or dry hair, then smoothed through – and it protects against damage from use of flat irons.

Testers say: 'A great product for my Mum's frizzy hair; it gave well-defined curls and looked in better condition overall; was very longlasting' • 'made my hair soft and shiny' • 'I was impressed by how smooth and glossy my hair looked, and it controlled my split

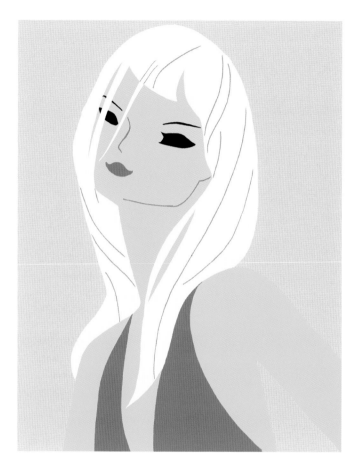

Testers say: 'I really liked this: not too runny; worked best first on towel-dried hair before blow-drying, then again before the straighteners – that gave a nice shiny look, and kept the frizz away' • 'easy to apply, and made my hair bouncy but smooth, with good shine. Excellent at defrizzing: easily the best I tried'.

Tommyguns Smooth & Finish Cream

 This is most appropriate for summer haircare: a jojoba oil-rich crème (it also features vitamin E) to nourish, strengthen and 'finish' summer hair. Great for adding 'definition' and texture, without flyaways, and boosting moisture and shine.

Testers say: 'Does exactly what it says it will! Compared well to my current product, so I would buy this one' • 'loved the sleekness it gave' • 'really helped with defrizzing and definitely made hair smoother – no problem with stickiness or lankness, as long as you didn't use too much' • 'very easy to comb through damp hair; my hair was certainly sleeker and smoother' • 'although I straighten my hair, it tends to go wispy and frizzy about midday but with this, it stayed poker straight and shiny!' • 'helped my hair go an extra day without a wash'.

ends' • 'really tamed flyaways – you only need a tiny bit, so it's good value' • 'my hair is so much smoother and sleeker if I apply this on damp hair, then style as usual'.

Lee Stafford Climate Control Serum (Step 3)

Another victorious product from Lee Stafford, the third step in his regime to conquer frizz, this smoothing potion interacts with the heat from a drier to 'melt into hair, creating a special film to protect hair from thermal damage'. It features the same Liquid Umbrella Technology™ as his Climate Control Protection Spray, opposite (the fourth step), but we trialled the products separately and they all excelled.

tried & tested
hair styling products

You're either a mousse or a gel person, when it comes to styling, so we recruited testers for specific 'hair panels' who really know what they're looking for in these products. Lots of high-street and affordable 'designer hair' ranges proved themselves shining stars in each category. For marvellous mousses, see here – and for gorgeous gels, flip the page.

Styling mousses

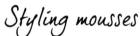

 Shockwaves Styling Plus
Conditioning Gloss & Body Mousse

 7.42/10 From the Shockwaves Styling Plus range, this contains pro-vitamin B5, to infuse hair with moisture and improve flexibility, while shielding against heat damage (from tongs, straighteners, etc). Flexible hold 'without crunchiness', they promise (and mousse-users will know what they're talking about!).

Testers say: 'Great nozzle, so no spurty spray all over the place; I applied it as directed, with a comb, and it worked well; hair was easy to style, smoother and less fuzzy, more body, and style lasted into the next day – a good result' • 'as long as you don't overdo the amount, it's not sticky' • 'works well: made my hair glossier – a bargain!' • 'smells pleasantly of green apples'.

 James Brown London
Volumising Mousse

 6.93/10 James Brown is one of the most sought-after session stylists in the world, loved by Sienna Miller, Lily Allen, Daisy Lowe and Kate Moss. However, his haircare range is very much targeted at mere mortals, price-wise – here, a simple body-building mousse with pro-vitamin B5, 'to give hair natural hold that you can still run your fingers through'.

Testers say: 'Hair seemed more glossy and salon-fresh; good volume; it pretty well delivers on the promises' • 'hair looked natural, not stiff, and there was a nice gloss' • 'my very fine, straight hair looked lighter but fuller; boosted the volume, and results lasted pretty well' • 'hair was fuller and styled more easily'.

Tommyguns Miraculous Volumising Thickening Mousse

 Does your hair lack volume, fullness and thickness? Is it fine, thin and difficult to style? Or baby-soft, with 'flyaways'? Tommyguns claim this mousse will meet those challenges, with strengthening, gloss-boosting ginseng, plus proteins to build hair volume.

Testers say: 'Worked well to lift fine hair prone to greasiness; definitely better than other budget mousses I have used' • 'gave my fine, shoulder-length hair much more body and the effects lasted five days! Hair looked much more streamlined and polished, smooth, and definitely brought out the colour'.

 Elvive Styliste Non-Stop Volume Mousse

This boosts hair volume, particularly – where it's most needed – at the roots. It's enriched with a special ingredient that L'Oréal call Expansyl-A®. (Oh, how we would love to be flies on the wall while they make these high-tech names up!)

 tip

'If you have "baby hairs" around the forehead which somehow defy styling, smooth them into place with an eyebrow brush (or toothbrush) spritzed with hairspray.' *Orlando Pita*

Testers say: 'I was impressed by how well it boosted volume, and stayed put after being styled; quite shiny too' • 'really liked the fruity scent' • 'I was impressed by the lack of residue' • 'my husband even commented on how good my hair looked – which he hasn't done for ages' • 'I let my hair dry naturally and it easily fell into a nice shape of its own accord – a miracle!'

John Frieda Luxurious Volume Thickening Mousse

Also rich in pro-vitamin B5, this features added heat-protection and is alcohol free. Part of a volume-boosting 'thickening' range from John Frieda, it's designed to make hair feel bouncier and fuller while delivering a flexible, natural hold.

Testers say: 'I was particularly pleased with the excellent lift and volume for fine, thick, flyaway hair' • 'good natural shine, no residue and longlasting results' • 'I've hated hair mousse for years, but this gave good body and hair stayed natural looking for about three days' • 'hair was more manageable; it boosted volume and lift: one of the best mousses I've tried'.

 Alberto V05 Styling Mousse Extra Body

 VO5's styling mousses feature UV filters to help protect hair from environmental damage; there are two options (the other is Mega Hold), but Extra Body – for volume and lift – is the one testers felt delivered the required va-va-voom.

Testers say: 'Made my hair very shiny and healthy looking; much better when I learnt not to use too much' • 'lovely scent of red apple; made my hair very easy to style; didn't feel crispy; looked shiny and healthy; full of bounce all day' • 'a friend asked what perfume I was wearing: it turned out to be my hair she could smell' • 'fulfilled all its promises: extra body lasted, there was volume, lift and longlasting hold – and no glueyness or greasiness'.

 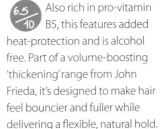

Styling gels

Like we say: you either love what gels do for your hair, or you don't. (They tend to deliver slightly stronger hold than mousses.) Panels of gel devotees trialled the entries in this category – and rated these most highly, from a wide field. But do remember, you only need the teeniest bit, worked up from the nape of your neck.

 L'Oréal Studio Line Indestructible Gel

 L'Oréal claim a 'technological innovation, style memorising effect' for this flip-top product which has been around for some time. They say it allows your style to 'bounce back' – and is 'hand, hood and helmet-resistant'. (The Boots website said it was 'helmut resistant', which gave us one of the best laughs in 18 months of working on this book.)

Testers say: 'Easy to apply; could run fingers up through it and it stayed like that; no stickiness; hair stayed in place all day – had some style memorising properties! If hair got windswept it would easily go back again' • 'my son, 20, thought this was quite effective with his thick, blonde hair – very useful if you're just coming up to a cut and want to look more groomed' • 'very easy to work with on my fine, long hair, which is dry at ends and oily at roots; was very shiny and style held all day – I would buy this' • 'gave good lift and lived up to manufacturer's promises'.

 Alberto Balsam Wet Look Styling Gel

 This is one for those after-that-catwalk-inspired 'wet' look. Non-sticky, it gives firm, longlasting hold – but also washes out without leaving a trace of greasiness. Better suited to short hair, or neat up-dos – can you imagine a wet-look mane? (We'd rather not.)

Testers say: 'Very easy to apply; gave that "just out of the shower" look – if that's what you want!' • very nice fruity smell; made fine hair very easy to manage and style held all day' • 'you need to use quite a lot for a wet look; otherwise just use it to tame top frizzies' • 'faint scent which I liked'.

Wella High Hair Crystal Styler

 More a 'setting lotion' than a gel – but not a mousse, so we've lumped it here. With heat-protective pro-vitamin B5 and UV filters – and the 'crystal' in the name alludes to its shine-boosting nature.

If you OD on hair gel, just wet the section of hair (or use a wet towel) to dilute the product a bit, and then style as normal.

Testers say: 'A great way to style my fine hair, masses of it, which has a slight wave, so will go either straight or curly with minimal encouragement. Worked best on clean, damp hair' • 'better than my usual product, which tends to leave curls crispy' • 'lovely and easy to apply; I used this every day when I blow-dried and it kept the sleekness and style very well' • 'improved the shine, and helped keep the style' • 'gave a nice shine, and really tamed my curl'.

 Alberto V05 Gel Spray Mega Hold

 Simply spritz this gel (yes, it has a slight identity crisis) on to the roots of towel-dried hair, before blow drying. The V05 styling range offers three gel options, of which this promises 'long-lasting, total control'. According to Alberto, it features an Aquascreen™ complex: a resin which absorbs less atmospheric moisture than traditional formulas, for greater resistance to humidity.

Testers say: 'My thick, coarse, dry hair was much easier to style and manage; gave a lot of lift by spraying it on the roots' • 'it fixed my hair for a period of time – but that's about it' • 'the plus is that you can use this on wet or dry hair' • 'the spray design means you can aim it into your roots' • 'flyaways improved, hair more "together"'.

Santé Styling Gel ❀❀

 For our more green-minded readers, good news that a product certified by the BDIH – the European natural standards board – made it in this category. No petroleum-based ingredients or synthetic preservatives – just hair-holding glycerine, birch extract, sorbitol, cellulose and xanthan gums (not as gummy as it sounds), and an algae extract.

Testers say: 'Silky gel, easy to apply; made my hair feel soft and smooth' • 'I found I could leave my hair to dry with gel in, then quickly brush it out with dryer on warm to remove gelled look but give a styled finish; held the style for about eight hours' • 'a fraction too much and it looked lank' • 'easily the best for styling my fine hair – excellent'.

Styling waxes

These aren't on everyone's shopping list, but for short and choppy hair styles they're a must: a little dab of wax warmed between the fingers and twizzled round hair ends defines cut and colour. Most waxes are steals, actually, so we had lots to try out. Now the bad news: not many put in a good performance, except these two – which most testers waxed lyrical about.

 Alberto V05 Styling Wax

Not much to say about this, except Alberto says it's ideal for shorter, cropped styles or flicked-out ends on longer, layered styles (in common with most waxes).

Testers say: 'This provided separation and texture with shine, on my thick but thinning hair; it was easy to apply and work through the hair, and the results lasted all day' • 'compared very well with my usual styling products; hair looked shinier, and felt nice and soft' • 'took away fluffiness

well; gave a shiny natural finish; good for long hair and fringes, too' • 'it was light and my hair still had room to move'.

John Frieda Luxurious Volume Thickening Texture Paste

 From the range targeted at all women who want 'bigger' hair: a non-sticky, lightweight professional formula which helps define both long and short styles, as well as taming flyaways. It contains sunscreen for added protection.

Testers say: 'This added a lot of texture and volume to my short, fine, feathered hair, and banished frizz and most flyaways; I thought this lived up to the promises' • 'wonderful that this soft wax tamed my hair, but left it looking voluminous and thick; SPF is a wonderful idea, and so practical' • 'completely lived up to the promises' • 'good shine with no hint of greasiness; made my hair appear much fuller and glossier' • 'on my mid-length hair this helped me to create volume' • 'nice to use and gave my hair a bit more "sturdiness"'.

tried & tested
hairsprays

Hairsprays are a love 'em or hate 'em styling product: some women won't set foot outside without a zhoosh; others find they instantly give 'helmet hair'. So we specifically recruited panellists for these hairspray trials who use them as part of their everyday styling regime. After much spritzing of many products, they identified quite a few spray 'steals' (and some SuperSteals, too), most of which additionally come in handbag sizes.

Wella System Professional Ultimation

 A sleek, tall, silver tube from Wella System Professional, which, they tell us, promises 'strong and flexible hold'. It's said to dry quickly and brush out easily (a major factor with hairspray), and to shield hair against the effects of humidity. Now for the science bit: the formula features 'nanoreflectors', which apparently 'transform light into radiant shine', and hair-strengthening vitamin E.
Testers say: 'Liked the large, funky packaging; the strong smell evaporated quickly; it gave a natural hold on my thick, long hair that lasted hours; not sticky at all; very impressed' • 'held style in my fine hair all day; fantastic hold which would be good for up-dos' • 'sprayed out in a light mist; very pleased that it held all night, even in strong wind and rain; loved this' • 'washed out the next day with no residue' • 'would recommend this to others with curly hair, as it gives hold without being "crunchy"; I was concerned this would add volume but it simply held my style and kept the frizz at bay!'

Toni & Guy Firm Hold Hairspray

super steal

7.14/10 Internationally renowned styling brand Toni & Guy explain that this delivers 'micro-fine lasting hold with flexibility to hair in need of control without stiffness'. Depressing the button certainly releases the most ultra-fine mist of style-setting ingredients, thereby avoiding another hairspray downside: a great clumpy wet bit, where you've targeted your first whoosh.
Testers say: 'This gives a perfect hold on my very thick, curly, hard-to-tame hair; spray a little from afar then add more gradually for a natural look' • 'my style stays perfect and looks even better the day after' • 'this enables me to do elaborate up-dos, or a straight style, and know they will be the same at the end of the evening' • 'finished effect is natural, flexible and lovely for my very difficult hair; kept my style all night in a club – I couldn't fault it' • 'user-friendly and left a shine'.

Lee Stafford Hold It Tight Firm Hold Barnet Hairspray

7.1/10 The range created by stylist Lee Stafford – who's won a slew of accolades, including Men's Hairdresser of the Year – has done very well in our trials. The bright pink packaging contains a spray that promises firm hold, but not stiffness. And, to our noses, this smells more pleasant than most.

Testers say: 'Incredibly easy to hold and use; consistent mist; finished effect felt firm but flexible; my fine, straight hair looked natural and healthy – remarkable!' • 'held my thick, coarse, frizzy hair beautifully, especially after straightening' • 'easy to brush out' • 'light and fine; never felt I was overloading my hair; gave a lovely sheen – I really liked this' • 'very good value – no downsides at all'.

  Tresemmé Salon Finish Extra Hold Hairspray

6.77/10 Tresemmé offer many different hairspray options, but the one our testers really liked – which comes in a giant 500ml can – is designed to provide all-day control with longlasting, extra-firm hold. They recommend using it not just for

tip

Even if you don't use hairspray, there's something you should know about spraying hair: it's a fantastic 'carrier' for fragrance. The late, great Estée Lauder used to recommend that women spray a 'cloud' of their favourite fragrance, and walk into it. It's a fabulous thing to do before an evening out, and every time you move your head, you get a whisper of your perfume. (And so does anyone who gets within nuzzling distance.)

fixing your style, but for extra volume: spray under the hair at the nape of the neck with your head flipped forward, then flip back and spray again from 10–12 inches away.

Testers say: 'Finished effect was natural looking and lasted a lot longer than I expected; brushed out very easily; very impressed with its stay-put quality' • 'I'm a hairspray addict and it took me a

long time to discover the "right" product – now I have!' • 'my fine, limp hair stayed put for quite a while and looked good' • 'gave a natural hold with some movement; even held all evening when I was dancing – impressive'.

John Frieda Luxurious Volume Thickening Hairspray

6.56/10 According to John Frieda, 7.7 million women in the UK 'suffer from fine, limp hair'. This va-va-voom-ifying sub-brand within the John Frieda collection spans everything from shampoo to styling products, with this quick-drying spray as a finale. It's been created to set styles fast while locking in volume, offering '24-hour soft, flexible hold'. It also contains sunscreen, to shield hair. Some testers loved this; others felt it gave too firm a hold.

Testers say: 'I was very impressed by this: normally I only spray my fringe, but soon I used this one all over, and it was very natural looking, but lasted all day' • 'came out evenly and in a light mist; looked pretty natural and flexible and my style lasted as long as I wanted it to, then brushed out easily' • 'did make my hair look thicker, and style held a bit longer too'.

tried & tested
hand cream

Mmm. We love hand creams. And you certainly adored these, which scored incredibly well – among dozens tried! – and are priced so reasonably you have no excuse for un-silky hands again. Ever. (We've included plenty, with lots of natural options for 'green' goddesses, too.)

 Dr. Organic Bioactive Skincare Manuka Honey Hand & Nail Cream ❁

 This very reasonably priced range from Holland & Barrett features some really delectable products. Our testers loved this, in its hefty tube, at an un-hefty price: a luxuriously-textured yet sinks-in-fast cream that is a must for honey-lovers, because of the straight-from-the-honey-jar smell as you squeeze it out.

Testers say: 'Very good on dry skin, especially "gardener's fingertips"; gave a good sheen to nails' • 'excellent overnight treatment under cotton gloves for my son's eczema; after three nights the patches had gone' • 'lovely, good-enough-to-eat honey smell; hands felt very soft and smooth; a fantastic hand cream, and great value; also worked well on dry knees'.

Liz Earle Naturally Active Hand Repair ❁

A 50ml tube of this, perfect for the handbag, comes in at under a tenner. That makes this the most expensive – per millilitre – hand cream in this category, but it's still a fraction of the cost of some luxury creams on the market and we felt it was worthy of inclusion, first, because it's a great product (we both love it) and secondly, for all the Liz Earle fans out there, who are legion. Light but velvety, it offers skin-strengthening echinacea and hops, moisturising B5, vitamin E and betacarotene; it's subtly aromatic, with bergamot, camomile, neroli and lavender.

Testers say: 'Excellent packaging; has a perfect consistency, rather like a Mr Whippy ice cream – smooth and silky to apply; hands felt incredibly smooth and nails benefited from regular use' • 'not oily, so I can open a door with a round handle – smells good and feels good; I really liked it' • 'works a treat; hands felt soft and silky' • 'skin felt in better condition and looked smoother; nails seemed to shine' • 'heavenly fragrance' • 'my hands look and feel great: my husband asked if I had been for a manicure'.

Organic Bloom by Skin Blossom Care and Protect Hand Cream ❁ ❁ ❁

A teensy, no-nonsense, Soil Association-certified organic brand, which punched above its weight with this shea-butter based cream, which also features grapeseed extract,

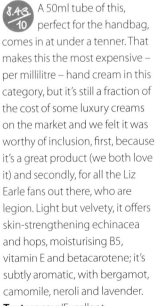

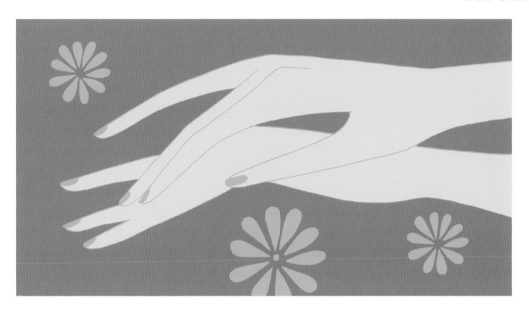

sunflower oil and is delicately scented with rose geranium.

Testers say: 'Lovely, clean geranium smell; very moisturising, and nails looked really good after' • 'lots of people in the office have commented on the smell – and been stealing it to use' • 'you only need a little: it goes in quickly and is fantastic for softening my hands' • 'really impressed by how quickly this product is absorbed' • 'relieved dry, wrinkled appearance immediately' • 'has kept eczema outbreaks on knuckles and between fingers at bay' • 'as an overnight treatment, this greatly improved my hands'.

 Neutrogena Norwegian Formula Hand Cream

 A real beauty classic. This cream's history starts with Norwegian fishermen: Neutrogena discovered that the oils in the fish they were handling had moisturising properties, and set about replicating them synthetically. It's a legendary barrier cream, especially useful in freezing weather, enriched with glycerine – and is available in Unscented (which we trialled) and Scented versions.

Testers say: 'Top marks! I am a long-term fan of this very thick cream, which improves dryness and rough skin round nails instantly, leaving hands soft and smooth' • 'a wonder cream and costs next to nothing; you only need a little dab and if you wash your hands in warm water first, the heat helps it spread' • 'works wonders for dry, chapped hands' • 'I have no age spots, which may be something to do with my long-term use of this product'.

 Beautifully Delicious Handluscious Honey & Almond Hand Lotion

 Like the Dr. Organic winner, above, this smells delectably honey-ish, and comes in a portable flip-top tube that's pretty handbag friendly. NB: we're quite amused that Beautifully Delicious have to put on the label: 'Warning: delicious but not edible'. Beware, though, if you don't like the smell of marzipan – as some of our testers did not.

Testers say: 'I liked the fact it was in a tube and easy to squeeze out the correct amount; it smoothed in and absorbed easily' • 'too large a tube to carry round, but great for your bedside table; really easy to rub in – loved the smell and it made my hands feel really moisturised; it also worked a treat on my feet before bed' • 'my hands were supersoft, and it smelt good enough to eat. I will decant it into smaller pots for bag/car/desk, etc'.

Tisserand Intensive Hand & Nail Cream ❋

 This jojoba-rich hand cream is free from synthetic fragrances, SLES and parabens, and also comes in a go-anywhere tube. Non-greasy, it has a soft, floral/spicy fragrance entirely derived from essential oils (geranium, orange blossom, rose, bergamot, camomile).

Testers say: 'This thick, smooth cream brightened my hands immediately without making

For a hand deep treat, slather them with an extra-thick layer of cream, slip on rubber gloves and do the dishes. The heat of the washing-up water is almost as effective at helping the cream penetrate as those heated mitts in expensive nail salons.

them shiny, or too slippery on the keyboard; the most effective hand cream for dry skin I have found – thank you!' • 'liked the light lavender smell, smallish tube – and it helped dry skin between my fingers, particularly' • 'liked the floral smell' • 'kept my hands thoroughly moisturised, and I had fewer incidents of broken or chipped nails after two weeks of using this product'.

 UMI Pomegranate & Acacia

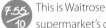 This is Waitrose supermarket's own-label range: a sleek, chic, silver plastic tube featuring shea butter and sweet almond oil, with the characteristically tangy scent of pomegranate – an ingredient that's rich in antioxidants.

Testers say: 'Generous size; chic packaging; light and non-sticky lotion, which smoothed in very

easily; I could resume typing and writing within ten seconds or so; very pleasant uplifting fragrance' • 'nice instant moisture boost, though not as hydrating as my more expensive one' • 'heavenly fruity, fresh smell; you find yourself putting it on just to smell it – very effective on dryness, but no noticeable effect on nails' • 'hands still soft and smooth the next day: I love this hand cream and would definitely buy it and recommend it' • 'quite a big tube but fitted into my handbag; perfect consistency, so moisturising I took it all the way up my arms – fabulous!'.

The Body Shop Almond Oil Daily Hand & Nail

 A blend featuring sweet almond oil (to replenish moisture and enhance suppleness), plus organic soya oil (rich in nourishing Essential Fatty

Acids), and Community Traded beeswax and shea butter. This is the 'sister' product to the nail strengthener/cuticle treatment that did so well in both those categories, and if you used both products diligently you would be on the fast-track to gorgeously groomed hands – no question.

Testers say: 'Ten or 11 or 12! Creamy, smooth product that soaked in brilliantly in seconds, which is one of my main criteria; helped dry cuticles – a lovely discovery that outshone my usual hand cream' • 'I even put cotton treatment gloves on overnight and my hands were very happy the next day' • 'is lasting me for ages – my hands are nice and soft and since the BUAV has certified there is no animal testing with The Body Shop products I might be persuaded to buy them again – this hand cream is just about good enough for me to consider it' • 'very practical and easy to carry round; love the smell; less greasy than my usual product – I would buy'.

Korres Honeysuckle Hand Cream SPF15 ❁

7.33/10 At the top end, price-wise, but it does feature a handy (sorry!) SPF15 – which is very relevant for hands, as they tend to pick up a lot of incidental sun damage (and are therefore vulnerable to age spots). Honeysuckle doesn't just smell pretty: it's soothing to sensitive skin, and the cream also offers vitamins B8 and B5 (to strengthen brittle nails), plus zinc oxide and vitamin E. Like all the Korres range, it screens out parabens, mineral oils, silicones and propylene glycol.

Testers say: 'Lovely, soft, creamy product; very easy to apply; great for use after handwashing, and good for night, when I put gloves on top – lovely, soft smell of honeysuckle flowers, not overpowering' • 'used regularly there is definitely an improvement in the appearance of my hands and nails; extremely moisturising: my hands look brilliant' • 'like the flip top, and really rapid absorption: hands look less careworn and dry, nails less brittle – great scent and had a really positive effect on my hands: they looked younger!'.

And a special mention for...

Yes to Carrots Pampering Hand Nail Spa

9.05/10 We thought you should know about this, even though it's not strictly a hand cream. It's an oily scrub (nicer than it sounds, trust us), which you smooth into hands, leaving them brighter – and super-soft. (Nice to use in the bath.) Our Beauty Steal panellists so loved it, we couldn't leave it out. (And you might also like to know that YTC's own hand cream – C a Softer You Hand & Elbow Moisturising Cream – is fabulous too, so it is well worth checking out, to use after you've scrubbed.

Testers say: 'Big pot makes it a luxury product for the bathroom; loved the (non-carroty) fragrance and hands felt wonderfully soft and smooth: my husband tried it and loved it too' • 'definitely worth a weekly treatment, made a big difference to softness of hands – they felt lovely after use' • 'bright, attractive packaging; from all the products I tested, I loved this the most – felt like luxury and I would definitely recommend it if you have dry hands' • 'made my skin feel soft as a baby's bum' • 'I don't normally use a hand scrub but will from now on!'.

how to blag
beauty freebies

Lack of the readies needn't mean doing without in the beauty arena. With a little knowhow, and a modicum of time and effort, you can look as high-maintenance as any lady who lunches...

Make-up: book in to your favourite brand/s at a department store for a free make-up or a new look. If you time it right, you can get all glammed up for a date – for nothing!

Fragrance: float in to your favourite perfume hall – and spritz! But beware you don't end up too much of a cocktail: three is plenty. If you're going out, stick to your favourite.

Skincare samples: if you're looking for something specific – day moisturiser, say, or night cream/serum – talk to a brand consultant and ask for a free sample of something suitable to try before you buy. Keep an eye out for product launches, when companies tend to sample heavily on lots of ranges, from skin- and suncare to fragrance.

Upkeep: ask your favourite hair salon, spa or beauty salon if they need models for training. You might get a free cut, colour (results not guaranteed!), facial, manicure or even a Brazilian bikini wax. NB: you'll probably need to be flexible, timewise.

Loyalty cards: sign up for all these moneypots and remember to bring them with you every time you buy – you can end up with lots of useful things for free.

Gifts with purchase (GWP): keep a beady eye on your favourite brand counters and ads in magazines, and beauty websites, but remember – only buy products you really want, not just anything because it happens to offer a GWP!

Barter: organise swap shops for products. Everyone gets to clear out the products that don't suit them and try a whole range of new ones.

Girls night in: give each other a mani/pedi, mini-back/neck/shoulder massage, or even a facial or blowdry. If you can't recruit a friendly beauty therapist to guide you through your paces (you could barter instruction for a meal, say, or shopping), take along a how-to beauty book – like one of ours! Be extra diligent and you could even find that you have a moneyspinner on your hands (and face, and feet…).

Enter competitions and draws: on our website, www.beautybible.com, we organise fantastic prize draws for every issue: no strings attached; just fill in a form and ping! (There are others, too.)

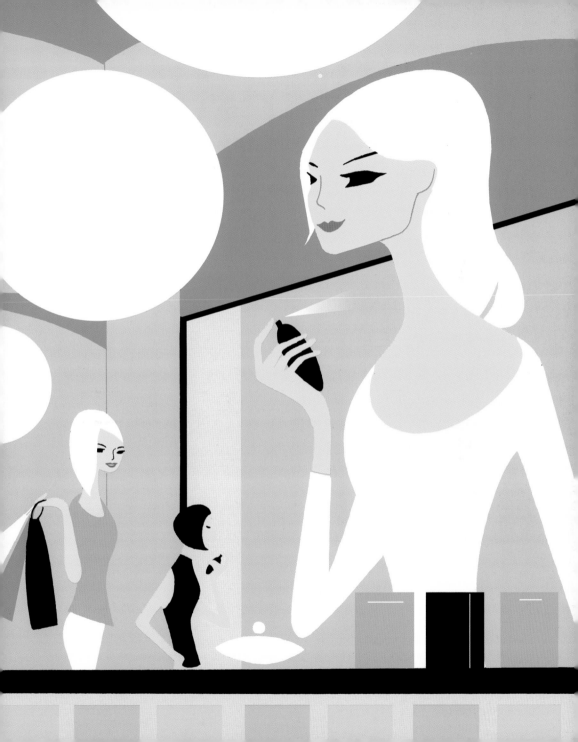

tried & tested

lip balms & treatments

You absolutely don't have to spend a fortune on lip balms and treatments – which is good news, because the best tip is to slip a little lip balm into the pocket of every jacket, to keep lips lusciously kissable, 24/7 – winter or summer. We tested dozens, including natural and 'green' options – many of which did really well: great scores, great products, great prices. So here are lots of options for you, with the top scorers so natural they're definitely good enough to eat.

Essential Care Organic Lip Silk ✿✿✿

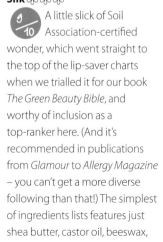

9/10 A little slick of Soil Association-certified wonder, which went straight to the top of the lip-saver charts when we trialled it for our book *The Green Beauty Bible*, and worthy of inclusion as a top-ranker here. (And it's recommended in publications from *Glamour* to *Allergy Magazine* – you can't get a more diverse following than that!) The simplest of ingredients lists features just shea butter, castor oil, beeswax, coconut oil, calendula extract, rosemary extract and orange essential oil – 100 per cent organic (and, we say, literally good enough to eat, which we personally feel is relevant with a lip balm, as most of it is ingested by mouth).

Testers say: 'Practical, dinky, twist-up tube, lovely on the lips; not sticky, just soft and soothing' • 'I'm trying to wean myself off Vaseline, because of the petrochemicals in it, so this product is very important to me' • 'applied at the first sign of chapping, this does the business' • 'I work in a dry office, so lip balm's essential' • 'looks easily as nice as the lip gloss I tested: gives a soft, sexy shine and great kissability…though further research needed'.

John Masters Lip Calm ✿✿

8.43/10 You'll find this in Jo's handbag (and several of her winter coat pockets): a twist-up stick of hydration, which is oh-so-subtly infused with vanilla, lime, tangerine and ylang-ylang. With extra virgin olive oil, shea butter, jojoba, kukui and wheatgerm, it also makes a great 'slick' of gloss over lipstick, Jo finds.

Testers say: 'I've tried many types of lip salve and this is by far the best natural one' • 'did exactly what it said on the box' • 'nice to have in your handbag and works very well' • 'my lips felt less dry, even when it was really cold' • 'prevented sore, chapped lips when I had a runny nose'.

Balm Balm Fragrance Free Lip Balm ❀ ❀ ❀

 If you eat organic food, you almost certainly want your lip balm to be equally pure – because it ends up in the same place. Balm Balm's products are multi-functional – you can also use this teeny pot of Soil Association-certified goodness on your face, heels – wherever (it's in all Sarah's bags and her stable). And this fragrance-free version is gentle enough even to use on new-borns, with just five ingredients (all organic): shea butter, sunflower oil, beeswax, calendula oil and jojoba oil.

Testers say: 'My lips are always soft now and look fantastic; it gives a natural-looking sheen' • 'blends in beautifully; silky rather than greasy; my lips felt instantly

softer, less cracked and much more comfortable. It eases cracked skin, too: I used it on my elbows and a small amount made my skin feel softer and absolutely sublime!' • 'nice to use, and I like one product that can do everything' • 'simple but good packaging' • 'softening effect on lips lasted well, and it was very good on other dry patches' • 'when I put this product on my nails, it made them look healthy and shiny, as if I'd applied a layer of nail varnish'.

Korres Guava Lip Butter ❀

 Korres chose guava fruit for this balm because it's rich in vitamin C and B vitamins.

tip

For a 'bee stung' look, apply lip balm lavishly and then pat on lipstick using your finger. Alternatively, create your own tinted lip balm with a lip pencil, swirling it first in the balm, then in the lipstick – and lastly, transferring the sheer colour to your lips.

(We're less sure why they choose to mention in their blurb that guava is also good for dyspepsia, or indigestion!) In a pot rather than a tube, this has a base of shea butter and rice wax; Korres also offer tinted versions, all of which our testers praised – but scored slightly behind this. Worth checking out the whole Lip Butter range, though, we'd say.

Testers say: 'Brilliant – tackled sore lips immediately; great flavour – creamy and sweet' • 'I always look for natural ingredients, as I eat a lot!' • 'super tube – no wastage' • 'my lips felt great afterwards; I loved this so much that when I thought I'd lost it I had a mini-panic' • 'made my lips fabulously shiny and I got several compliments'.

W7 Vitamin E High-Moisture Aloe Vera

Congrats to W7 for getting three winners from their range of balms into this book (and we trialled literally dozens); one of them also did well as a lip-plumper, on page 120. Unprepossessing packaging, but good performance for this (non-natural) balm, which delivers the lip-quenching power of aloe vera.

Testers say: 'Not sticky at all, and solved my chapped/dry lip problem, despite what I might call dubious ingredients for something you eat (petrolatum and colourings); this is one of the few lip moisturisers that worked quickly and effectively when my lips were particularly dehydrated and sore' • 'tasted a bit chemical, but such great results I was prepared to put up with it' • 'gave a nice sheen to my lips, and used for a month has certainly improved the condition' • 'loved this and wouldn't be without it'.

Neal's Yard Remedies Organic Lip Formula ❀ ❀ ❀

 Another option, if you want something that's literally good enough to eat on your lips. One of Neal's Yard's first products to be certified organic, it offers soothing and healing calendula, comfrey and lavender, with skin-toning lemon and myrrh, in a protective and vitamin-rich soya oil, wheatgerm, sunflower and beeswax base.

Testers say: 'I can't fault this: my lips are definitely in better condition – lovely citrus aroma, and a good base for lipstick' • 'my builder son and his mates say it's brilliant for their chapped lips' • 'I'm going to throw out all my other lip balms and only use this nourishing product' • 'as always,

Neal's Yard produce quality for a very reasonable price'.

 e.l.f. Therapeutic Conditioning Balm

A little twist-up tube of subtly tinted balm, the shade our testers had was Strawberry Crème – a baby pink which isn't as baby pink on the lips, but is as strawberry crème scented! This balm offers a shielding, soothing blend, infused with vitamins A and E, plus shea butter, but it's primarily petroleum based.

Testers say: 'Fantastic: I loved this balm – light, velvety, lipsmackingly good, smelt of yum strawberry; instant relief for my chapped lips – am already converted – what a bargain!' • 'good, clear, subtle colour, with really good levels of moisture, which lasted several hours; one of the best tinted lip salves I have tried' • 'neat, practical – though not glamorous – packaging; felt lovely on my very dry lips. I wouldn't like to have a balm-free day – I am addicted to the stuff' • 'a very good product for a ridiculously cheap price' • 'my lips felt really soft after using this, though it needed reapplying every two hours or so'.

 W7 Vitamin E Soothing Menthol Lip Balm

 Breath-freshening menthol – which we find has a slight tingling effect – is the ingredient unique to this product, within W7's ultra-affordable range of five petroleum-based (ie, not natural) balms.

Testers say: 'Very creamy and comfortable to use: really moisturising – I would recommend this' • 'slightly minty, pleasant taste; moisturised well; didn't need to apply as often as my usual balm; I never thought anything would replace my good old Vaseline, but I would definitely buy this: great product' • 'fabulous; softened my lips incredibly well and was a little addictive!' • 'didn't last long on my lips but I loved the excuse to re-apply – one of the best balms ever, and the first I have used up totally'.

 Vaseline Intensive Care Aloe Vera Lip Therapy

 Vaseline Lip Therapy is a beauty classic – but our testers preferred this little green tin (which features soothing and hydrating aloe) to the original Vaseline-based formulation, which creates a barrier on lips

we love

with petroleum jelly. About as much of a 'steal' as a product ever gets, this.

Testers say: 'Perfect little pot; gorgeous smell; slight flavour; my lips are so much softer – the best lip moisturiser on the market' • 'good sturdy packaging – and now not a chapped bit in sight!' • 'liked the slight lemony taste' • 'very moisturising, and lip condition has improved; less flaky and dry' • 'not too greasy and didn't slide off after eating or drinking; not sticky or tacky; happy to see that the main ingredient was petroleum jelly' • 'the one thing you take to a desert island – I bought two dozen of these little pots of magic for friends' Christmas stockings'.

Balance Me Hydrating Rose Otto & Shea Butter Lip Balm ✽

 7.43/10 We're very fond of this little natural beauty brand, created by an ex-Lancôme PR. This tube of balm has a useful slanted dispenser, which makes for comfortable application of ultra-nourishing sweet almond oil, shea butter and beeswax – infused with fragrant rose otto and palmarosa – on to lips.

Testers say: 'Very pretty packaging, and easy to squeeze a

Oh, too numerous to mention. We're addicted, and not ashamed to say so. John Masters, Neal's Yard, Balance Me – all mentioned here – plus Dr. Organic 100% Organic Vitamin E Lip Balm, from Holland & Barrett's natural range. Oh, we nearly forgot! – our very own Beauty Bible Lip Balm, a chunky, pink (of course!) swivel-up stick of natural deliciousness, with shea butter, vitamin E and aloe vera, which seems to be becoming a cult item at a real 'steal' price – (only from www.victoriahealth.com).

little out of the soft plastic tube; felt very nice on my lips and sank in quickly; smells and tastes like roses, very pleasant – Turkish delight without the sickly sweet taste; my lips are very smooth and soft, even in horrid cold weather' • 'really impressed with this product; love the natural ingredients, and the smell is divine – lent it to a friend to fix his dry lip problem, and he is clinging to it' • 'bearing in mind how much lip product I eat, I'm very keen on natural products like this; I would definitely buy it, and it's pretty enough to make lovely little gifts, too'.

Kiehl's Lip Balm

 7.12/10 Not many Kiehl's products are going to limbo under our price ceiling, but

we're pleased to see this true beauty classic making a well-deserved appearance. Beauty editors and make-up pros have long sworn by this handbag-friendly tube of lip-soother, which contains skin-quenching squalene, and has a fairly paltry (but better-than-nothing) SPF4.

Testers say: 'Loved the classic Kiehl's retro packaging; definitely improved the condition of my lips' • 'really made a difference from the first night I used it; no dry lips in the morning' • • 'very moisturising – fine lines and dryness have disappeared' • 'lips softer, smoother and looked plumper; a little goes a long way' • 'very comfortable, not too greasy, and thankfully no flavour or smell'.

tried & tested
lip pencils

If you don't use a lip pencil, you're missing a (lip) trick. They help colour stay put, and, with their waxy texture, help prevent lipstick 'bleeding'. Here are some lipliners at prices guaranteed to put a smile – as well as some contouring colour – on your lips.

GOSH Velvet Touch Waterproof Lip Liner

 7.38/10 This is packed with pigments, and turns out to be 100 per cent waterproof. (We love waterproof.) At the same time, it's soft textured and fairly creamy, giving the 'velvet' finish its name implies. There are ten shades, but, as ever with lip liners, we advise choosing a shade that is as close to your natural lip tone as possible: the nudey, neutral Nougat Crisp that our testers tried ticks that box perfectly.

Testers say: 'The easiest lip liner I have ever tried: very easy to apply precisely; didn't drag; great colour and easy to smudge slightly without the line disappearing – would most

definitely buy' • 'very natural looking – unlike other lip liners I've tried; very good with a gloss on top' • 'I would give this ten-plus! Effortless to apply, lovely texture – the smoothest pencil I've ever used; no dragging, just lovely even colour with no fuss and no crumbly bits' • 'goes – and stays – exactly where it's put. Gives a totally realistic look – none of that awful panto effect, where the

outline stays put when everything else has worn off your lips' • 'the find of the year: stroke all over your lips, add a touch of gloss and you have a lip colour that lasts all day!'.

myface.cosmetics Lip Pencil

 7.3/10 Myface is the brand started by John Frieda's clever business partner Gail Federici, who was key to the global success of that brand (and John is a sleeping partner in this too). Add to that combo the talents of make-up pro Charlotte Tilbury, and no wonder the range is a 'wow' (we rate it highly). Cleverly, they categorise products by skintone, with three pencils for Fair skins, three for Medium, three for Dark, to take the guesswork

♡ *we love*

Jo recently picked up a trick from Lulu, which is to use two shades of lip liner to customise the perfect, lip-matched shade. She uses two 'lovely, soft-textured' products by myface.cosmetics from the 'Fair' collection, one of which did so well with our testers here.

out of shade selection. Our testers had Fair Nude, in this soft-textured pencil.

Testers say: 'Lovely product, my favourite of all – the first lip pencil that looked natural and stopped any "bleed"' • 'brilliant colour, really easy to apply, beautiful texture – it's quite moisturising, so I used the pencil as lipstick, and liked the result' • 'very easy to be precise; made my lipstick last a lot longer than normal – also lip glosses; great texture, which gave excellent definition to my ageing lips – great product' • 'good texture, nice and firm, but not too hard' • 'creamy, delightful texture, even at room temperature during horrible winter months; I would have given it top marks if it had been easier to sharpen'.

Revlon ColorStay Lipliner

 The name – Colorstay – says it all. This is Revlon's Duracell-bunny-of-a-range, designed to stay put for longer. (Ideal for summer or VIP events such as a wedding, but many women just wear it year round.) It contains a complex called SoftFlex™, as well as vitamin E and aloe for lip-conditioning, and 'sets' on the lips in minutes for that extended wear. Eight shades, and Nude was ours. It's twist-up, so it doesn't need sharpening.

Testers say: 'Twist-up pencil, making it really easy and quick to line my lips fully; went on smoothly and only needed very light pressure' • 'lasted longest as a base with lipstick, rather than clear gloss' • 'gave my thin lips better definition; far easier to apply and looked better than I imagined' • 'I drew a lovely precise line that really emphasised the shape of my lips, though I needed practice! I am really pleased with this product; I wouldn't normally buy a lip liner, but having seen how this lovely natural colour defines and shapes my lips, I will definitely be repurchasing' • 'loved the outline that this gave my lips – left them really pronounced and lush looking'.

Vie at Home Within Limits

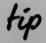 Something different, this, from the brand formerly known as Virgin Vie. This twist-up wax product is invisible: you glide the silky formula around your lips, where it acts as a barrier to keep your lipstick in check, preventing feathering, while reducing the appearance of fine lines. Our testers also liked it as an all-over base for lippie.

Testers say: 'A coloured lipliner can look artificial but I liked this, and my lipstick stayed in the right place, and lasted longer' • 'piece of cake to use; I made small feathery strokes round my mouth – very carefully, as I am not used to a lip pencil at all; made my lips feel really moisturised, and lipstick went on very evenly and easily. I really like it' • 'made my lipstick last through a cup of coffee, which is good – at 54 I have some lines round my lips: I was impressed with this and it's small enough to keep in my bag with my lipstick for reapplying' • 'I do feel safe with Virgin Vie, as I have been very pleased with the products I have used previously' • 'this was one of the best products you sent me'.

tip

Linda Evangelista – who Jo has interviewed in New York – has this to say: 'I don't do lipstick. I think lip liner and a slick of gloss give a much more modern and plumping effect. And my best trick is always to do my make-up in natural light: I keep all my make-up on a huge mirrored tray and I just take it to whatever window is looking good that day.'

lip gloss

Some truly outstanding scores for the 'steal' brands in this mood-lifting category. But be warned: there are plenty of others out there which our testers found tasted cheap, dried their lips or disappeared almost before they'd put the cap back on. So we say: read our testers' lips…

Revlon Super Lustrous Lip Gloss

8.5/10 We'd trialled this before, way back, but Revlon re-submitted it and our testers loved it (perhaps partly due to the sexy packaging). Of the eight shades, testers had a very wearable Nude Lustre.

Testers say: 'Ten out of ten! 'I'd given up on lip glosses but

---

tip

Sticky, cheap glosses can be a pig to remove. A make-up artist's tip is to swipe lips with a damp washcloth dipped in olive oil. (Great for eradicating any lip product, too – even dark lipstick.)

Revlon has converted me' • 'glossy, glam, tastes amazing, moisturising, colour lasted well, wonderful shimmery look, easy to apply with wand, everything you want' • 'looks like you've applied a nude lippy then gloss on top – gorgeous!'.

 Rimmel Volume Booster Lip Plump Gloss

7.94/10 We probably should have tested this under lip plumpers, but it got sent out as a regular gloss. No matter: testers liked it as a lip-shiner in its own right, trialled in 072 Rumour – one of a dozen shades.

Testers say: 'Great product! Love the subtle, pretty, natural-looking colour; lovely gloss that didn't feel heavy or sticky – had lots of compliments' • 'applicator brush is good, and the gloss made my

lips look fuller – would definitely buy it' • 'really comfortable to use, took well to my lips, not drying, colour deepens after a few minutes; boyfriend commented on how nice my lips looked – a good sign!' • 'I try to buy 80/20, natural/chemical: this would get in the 20!' • 'glossy but not greasy; nice subtle colour that anyone could wear – got any spares?!'

 Collection 2000 Love Your Lips Balmgloss

7.5/10 This is lip-conditioning as well as glossing, with vitamins, antioxidants, rosehips, apricot kernel, mango and grapeseed extract – plus SPF20. A perfect summer gloss, then, in six fruit-inspired shades (our mob got peachy-toned Darling 5). Like the Rimmel gloss, this has a small brush, not a sponge wand.

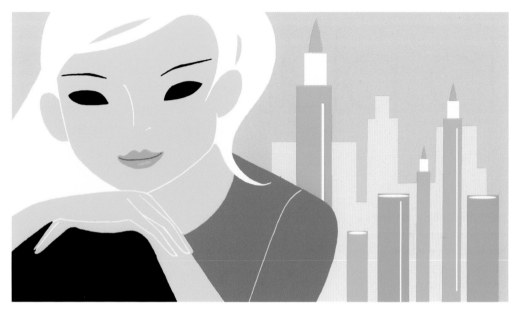

Testers say: 'Very glossy and glam – sheer, shimmery finish – fab! Easy to apply precisely' • 'not too thick, perfect for both day and night wear, with tiny particles of glitter that catch the light and give it a hint of glamour' • 'cute little brush' • 'colour looked very red/pink but was subtle on'.

 Maybelline Watershine Gloss

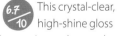 **6.7/10** This crystal-clear, high-shine gloss features 'natural water droplets derived from aqua-botanicals' (Maybelline-speak)'. Quite fruitily scented, initially, but worth a shot for anyone who finds some lip

glosses too sticky. Pale sheer pink 103 Crystal Rocks – our testers' 'homework' – is one of 15.

Testers say: 'Lovely and glossy, shimmery and very sheer: angled flexible wand makes application really easy, leaves my lips lovely and soft' • 'packaging is glam, and gloss goes on really nicely, with a good wand; instantly pepped up my appearance – good pick-me-up if you're looking a bit tired' • 'very glossy and made my lips look very slick, moisturised my lips and definitely no dryness – but did wear off quite quickly' • 'one of the least sticky glosses I've used' • 'I was impressed with the quality balanced with the price'.

 W7 Glamorous Gloss

 6.55/10 From this very inexpensive brand, offering lots of 'funky shades', our testers had deep, frosted burgundy Cherry Fizz.

Testers say: 'Liked this a lot: gave me very glam, glossy, gorgeous lips; very nice shade – sheer but still colourful, very sparkly' • 'the taste was nice' • 'easy to apply with the wand' • 'left my lips feeling moisturised, was like a colour wash – I liked it very much' • 'very subtle colour, even though it looks stronger in the tube; excellent find' • 'incredibly generous size of tube'.

tried & tested
lip plumpers

Do they really work? Give you a Pamela Anderson/Angelina Jolie pout? Well, not quite – but we were quietly impressed (and often amused) by our testers' reports on these affordable pout-boosters.

The 'lip-plumping' category embraces glosses, balms and lipsticks. Whatever the format, the questions Beauty Bible poses when sending out these products specifically relate to their lip-boosting effect, which can be real, though temporary – thanks to warming/tingly ingredients such as capsicum, cinnamon or ginger, which dilate blood vessels – or attributable to optical illusion, thanks to clever use of ingredients.

 Rimmel Volume Booster Lipgloss

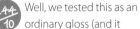 **7.44/10** Well, we tested this as an ordinary gloss (and it made it to our list of award winners, see page 118). Then, in another shade (012 Outrage), it did awfully well for its stated purpose as a 'lip plump' treat, too. The pout-boosting action is said to be down to marine collagen spheres and hyaluronic 'biospheres' to enhance volume and hydration, leaving lips smoother – both instantly, and over time. 'Up to 40 per cent fuller-looking lips', they promise. **Testers say:** 'Ten out of ten! It's not overly sticky, makes lips look fuller immediately – and moisturises: I love everything about it' • 'on first application, the tingling lasted about five minutes, then got less every time, now practically nonexistent' • 'lovely peachy-colour, very

natural looking' • 'lips looked smoother and fuller; the sparkly colour helps' • 'liked the simple packaging and subtle fragrance'.

 W7 Vitamin E Plumping High Moisture & Soften Lips

 7.10/10 W7 (a brand born in London W7) are a bit skimpy with info on their products, but this is a really inexpensive, sheer, glossy lip balm, featuring antioxidant vitamins and a 'top secret ingredient'. (We can't figure it out, although it does feel minty and cooling. No matter: these testers' comments say enough…) **Testers say:** 'I thought it would be rubbish from the packaging but it is super: I almost panicked when I couldn't find it one day' • 'very moisturising; made my lips so soft, they looked more youthful' • 'not certain of the plumping, but an excellent moisturising balm' • 'made lips slightly glossy; pleasant fragrance; stays for good amount of time' • 'I liked the SPF15'.

Prestige Wonder-Full Lip Plumping Gloss

 A curvy tube of lip-plumping gloss with what Prestige refer to as 'Maxi Lip™ technology. It works instantly – they call it a 'fabulously refreshing pain-free tingle' – and also contains ingredients which they claim will create a 'sexy bee-stung pout and encourage lasting fullness'. Our testers wore Chic, one of eight shades.

Testers say: 'Lovely. I was very impressed: gorgeous glossy colour shot with shimmer gave the illusion of fullness without pain (some lip plumpers hurt!)' • 'I noticed the tingle but no extra plumpness – my boyfriend said my lips did look plumper, so maybe it's all in the eye of the

we love

Actually, Jo doesn't: the fullness of her lips doesn't bother Jo (she's too busy worrying about stubby lashes). Nor does Sarah, though a bit of gloss always seems to have an effect.

beholder?' • 'if anything makes your lips look fuller and more 3D, it's the serious amount of glitter in this thick, shiny gloss' • 'smells of hazelnuts/choc, but tastes more cinnamony, with a hint of mint – OK at first, but on repeated wearings slight eau de car freshener' • 'I enjoyed the fresh sensation, but anyone who doesn't like sticky glosses might feel irritated – I don't mind, as it stops me grazing' • 'easy to apply with sponge-tipped applicator; gloss leaves high shine; lips smooth and a little plumped'.

tip

Troubled by lip gloss/lipstick marks on drinking glasses? Discreetly licking your glass before drinking from it prevents any unsightly smears! (We think the key word here is 'discreetly'!)

Time Delay Skin Treatments Instant Lip Plumper

It would be easy to be put off by the colour of this in the tube: a sort of shimmery coppery brown (there's just one shade). But on the lips, it's magically transformed into a wearable, universally flattering neutral with a high-gloss, volume-enhancing appearance. It tingles slightly (that's the capsicum), and contains nourishing ingredients which they promise will make 'lips look plumper day by day'.

Testers say: 'Perfect sponge applicator, and it certainly worked – an incredible lip plumping effect: gave a great look and I loved it; so did my teenage daughters, who thought the bee-sting feeling was worth the plumping!' • 'I liked the subtle sparkle effect, which made my lips look slightly fuller, they appeared less lined, though not dramatically bigger – I don't recommend kissing anyone while the tingle lasts on this!' • 'gave lips a nice appearance and a slight illusion of fullness; loved the colour and ease of application, also the tingle – so would buy, despite the lack of "pout"' • 'very strong spearmint fragrance made my mouth feel fresh'.'

tried & tested
lipstick

Here, you'll find the more common-or-garden type of lippy, with longlasting over the page. To be honest, the scores for these didn't rival the glosses we trialled. But we've identified these winners – all of which we'd be happy to have in our kit – among dozens of options out there, many of which taste as cheap as they are, our testers report.

M&S Autograph Sheer Gloss Lipstick

 Actually halfway between a gloss and a lipstick, this glamorously packaged slimline lippie has a super-soft texture. Of the 12 shades available, we tried Dusky Pink, a mid-rose.

Testers say: 'Very lovely colour; matt finish with a slight sheen; quite moisturising – and lasted ages, even through a greasy spag bol' • 'it's very slightly sheer, and not shiny, despite the name; the slanted shape makes it easy to apply; nicely moisturising' • 'I liked the design: it looked luxurious and different – a nice, slim, shiny metal casing; left my lips quite moisturised' • 'smooth and easy to use, very comfortable, not at all sticky and lasted quite well' • 'I like M&S products anyway and I would buy this'.

L'Oréal Colour Riche Shine Gelée Lipstick

 This 'nourishes with moisture like a balm and shines like a gloss', explain L'Oréal – but it certainly looks like a lipstick to us (trialled by testers in 102 Sugar Rose, a sheer-ish, candy-ish pink). You can feel the comforting shea butter; there's royal jelly, too, to condition lips. It has a light-reflective, shimmeringly pretty finish.

Testers say: 'Very creamy and moisturising; not much staying power, but I did like the feel and smell' • 'feels very rich and slippy; gives a glossy-to-sheer wash of colour rather than a precise line' • 'loved the smell, like sweet roses' • 'very comfortable on my lips, and feels good even after some time; my lips look lovely dressed in this, which is really easy to apply precisely, with or without lip liner' • 'not a shade I would normally wear, but it brightens up my face; practical case, and I love the coppery colour' • 'full of

If you find lippy leaves your lips dry, apply balm at least ten minutes before and let it sink in. Voilà – luscious lips!

moisture; very comfortable; neat packaging'•'went on well and evenly; lasted well'.

Barbara Daly Make-Up Lipstick

 This has a clever 'square edge' – a sophisticated bevelled shape which Barbara designed to allow for more accurate application. It comes in a velvet-finish black tube, and is available in 16 lip-flattering shades; our testers trialled soft-pink Sorbet.

Testers say: 'Lovely, light, very moisturising texture; looks sheeny and quite sheer – almost a glaze; the packaging is basic, but the lovely texture more than compensates'•'easy to apply and follow lipline; lips didn't feel dry at all; packaging is lovely, with soft lines and easy-click opening and closing'•'I wouldn't have bought this colour from looking at it, but it so brightened my face'•'I love this soft, satiny lippy; fabulous quality, good colour coverage, but not heavy; I'm so pleased I was given this to test. Excellent!'

GOSH Velvet Touch Lipstick

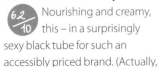 Nourishing and creamy, this – in a surprisingly sexy black tube for such an accessibly priced brand. (Actually,

we love

Jo's favourite lipstick 'steals' are somewhat numerous (as with glosses), and include the super-creamy myface Gigabyte Lipsticks in Strawberry Fields and Raspberry Sorbet, and the lip-quenching Maybelline Moisture Extreme range, which has SPF15 as a bonus.

the packaging for this Danish brand reminds us of the Nars range.) Don't be deceived by the colour in the tube: most of our testers had 134 Darling, which looks like a sad beige but goes on very sheer and pretty, with a hint of shimmer if it catches the light. (One tester got 122 Nougat instead, which she loved to bits.)

Testers say: 'A pleasant surprise: I like everything about this, including the colour – now one of my favourites'•'nice, smooth, creamy texture; easy to apply without lip brush; left lips moisturised and stayed on for a while; looked natural – I would buy'•'nice, light lipstick, but creamy enough to keep lips moisturised'•'easy to apply – I'm

not very good at it, but this seemed to follow the contours of my lips effortlessly; perfect colour, and people say it makes my face look brighter'•'I have already bought the matching lipliner'.

 e.l.f. Moisture Care Lip Colour

What an interesting product! Not only does this qualify as a SuperSteal (like all the ultra-affordable Eyes, Lips, Face range), but it's not like anything we've ever seen before: it comes in a see-through tube, like a lip gloss, with a sponge applicator that dispenses the very moisturising formula (which is definitely not a gloss). They call it a 'liquid lipstick' – and really, that's exactly what it is. Slightly coconutty taste, with a somewhat cooling action; our shade was pale pink Baby Lips, one of eight.

Testers say: 'Love this soft sheeny, natural-looking product, which is great for teens – and grown-ups! Would I buy? Yes' •'glossy and very moisturising; certainly had the pleasure factor; good packaging, in that you could see how much was left' •'great shade for everyday' •'staying power OK; lasted through a couple of cups of tea' •'liked the coconutty smell'.

tried & tested
longlasting lipstick

This category was a bit disappointing, with some appalling scores (at all price points) lagging behind these rather more impressive winners. Because long-lasting lipsticks can so often be drying, we've also included a definitive how-to from Bobbi Brown, to make your regular lipstick go the distance, *opposite*.

Max Factor Lipfinity

7.5/10 Max Factor have reigned supreme over this category for some time, and their beauty boffins are always working to upgrade the formulations of Lipfinity products. This incarnation is a two-step/two-product process: first, a lip 'paint' which is applied with a sponge applicator (and 'sets' in 60 seconds), then a glossy, almost shimmery Lipfinity 'balm' topcoat, to add a dewy finish without dissolving the colour. The Lipfinity products use a technology called Permatone™, an ingredient which 'provides semi-permanent colour by gently attaching colour pigments to the lips in a flexible mesh effect'. The result, they promise, is eight-hour colour, and Lipfinity comes in 24 shades (ours was 016 Glowing, a browny pink).

Testers say: 'First a creamy liquid that glided on very smoothly, then was slightly sticky as it dried; lips a little dry until I applied the light, balm-like gloss; then they were very soft and comfortable. Needed reapplying after six hours' • 'after a drink, the colour was fine and I just reapplied the top coat' • 'good that the colour never smudges out of the lips, or bleeds' • 'the colour stays, but you do need to moisturise your lips first, as it is drying' • 'lasted seven hours, through a heavy evening of birthday celebrations – I just applied the gloss twice to keep my lips soft looking' • 'I received so many compliments!'

Revlon ColorStay Mineral Lipglaze

 As you can tell by now, make-up with extra staying power is a special focus of Revlon, who have introduced a super-glossy entry to the longlasting lip category: a 'cushiony' formula with a mineral complex to condition lips, delivering luminous colour. Our testers enjoyed trialling a shimmering deep pinky-brown – 530 Infinite Rose.

Step-by-step to longer-lasting lip looks

From our make-up genius friend Bobbi Brown…

1 Buff lips with a wet flannel to remove flakes.

2 Apply balm, if your lips are dry – and let it soak in for a few minutes.

3 Outline lips with a lip pencil, and then 'colour in', using the same pencil.

4 Apply lipstick with a lip brush. (This gives a richer finish, rather than a sheer look, but it's a must if you want to enhance staying power – and always, for darker and bright lipstick shades.)

5 Place a tissue between your lips and press them together.

6 Reapply, using the brush.

7 DON'T add gloss, if you really want your lipstick to stay put; the shinier the finish, the faster it's likely to disappear.

Testers say: 'Lovely, silky-smooth texture; very moisturising: feels lovely on – I applied it before a meal and drinks that lasted seven hours; the lippie stayed the whole time; when I got home I could still see it' • 'very easy to apply with wand applicator, very moisturising and comfortable – not at all drying – really good finish' • 'I would definitely buy this: the colour is subtle and fairly natural – made my teeth look whiter, and I got compliments! Longlasting-wise, this lived up to 80 per cent of its promises – it was just as it had been after one drink, but after several, plus a meal, it needed reapplying' • 'lovely lip gloss – not sticky, and a really lovely colour; it lasted longer than regular lip gloss – but not that much' • 'this product stayed on much better than I thought it would – certainly beyond the first drink; I would never have thought of buying this brand, so it's nice to be proved wrong!'

cheap tricks
from very clever girls

Along the way, we've been lucky enough to pick up some great tips from fellow beauty editors and experts – who've tried everything, done everything, experimented with every type of gunk under the sun. Here are some of our favourites.

Newby Hands, beauty director, *Bazaar*: 'Facial massage is the single most important thing that I do. I always notice the difference if I get lazy. Anything that goes on your face, apply it upwards and outwards, using deep movements, really working the product into the skin and moving the flesh, from chin to temples. And it's free!'

'Dry shampoo is really good on baby-fine hair: spritz it on and leave in for added volume'

Catherine Turner, beauty director, *Easy Living*

Nicola Moulton, beauty director, *Vogue*: 'Smile at the mirror while you put on your blusher: it shows you the apples of your cheeks – and you see yourself smiling, which is such a lovely way to start the day.'

Yanar Alkayat, www.greenmystyle.com: 'My best tip is to put a couple of drops of oil into your regular daily moisturiser. I do the rounds: I like any Neal's Yard Remedies oil, or Aromatherapy Associates, but rosehip seed oil is my favourite: a miracle healer – a wonder oil.' (Look out for A'kin's version, on page 74.)

Karena Callen, former beauty director of *Red*, *Marie Claire* and other leading magazines: 'When I use fake tan, I dry myself with a hairdryer all over! But funnily enough, it only works with inexpensive fake tans, for some reason.'

Liz Earle, skincare guru: 'If you're on a strict budget, the skincare essentials are a cleanser and a moisturiser: buy other products as a treat, or ask for them as gifts.'

Kathy Phillips, international beauty director for Condé Nast Asia, and founder of This Works and Good Works: 'If I was stuck with no moisturiser, I would just use

And our own fave beauty tips

'When you're doing your face, do your lips, brows and cheeks first, then eyes last, to get the balance right'

Edwina Ings-Chambers, beauty director, *Sunday Times Style*

Jo: 'Once you've discovered a foundation brush (see page 8), there's no going back. It's the best investment in a flawless face you can make: you slap the stuff on and pat it into skin with the brush, using feathery tapping motions – and provided you've got the right shade of foundation, it looks utterly flawless.' (Or, if you're Sarah, dip the brush into the foundation and apply titchy amounts only where needed.)

Sarah: 'I love what supermodel Lauren Hutton once told me: as the years creep on, use less make-up better. It's much cheaper and you look far more gorgeous. I use titchy amounts of base, blusher, mascara, eyeliner and lippy, but take much more time and care applying them. Also get into body scrubs and dry skin body brushing: simply the best way to keep skin smooth, help it lap up body lotion – and prevent cellulite!'

almond or coconut oil on my face, neck and cleavage, and olive oil on my body.'

Marcia Kilgore, founder of Soap & Glory: 'Mix a little lemon juice with witch hazel (in a ratio of 1:4) to purge congested pores; soak a cotton ball and wipe over affected areas. And mix a dab of sun prep into your hand cream!'

Jo Glanville-Blackburn, beauty editor, *Woman and Home*: 'For me, details make all the difference: nails can be bare but always nourish your cuticles; groom your hair – even curls looks more beautiful when smoothed; and perfect skin with the sheerest coat of foundation, to even out blemishes and mottled skin. You will instantly look more

effortlessly groomed, which just makes every busy day a little easier.'

Barbara Daly, make-up artist: 'Always do your make-up in bright daylight, if possible. And don't get stuck in a make-up groove: book free makeovers from brands that appeal to you. You'll learn what you like – and what you don't. But only buy if you really love a product: otherwise, walk away, saying sweetly that you want to consider it.'

Rosie Green, beauty director, *Red*: 'A tiny dab of iridescent powder on the inner corners of the eyes makes you look younger, prettier and more wide awake.'

tried & tested
mascaras

We always say the same for mascaras: we want no clumping, no smudges, no flakes – and no sore eyes, please. Happily, the mass market has some very impressive choices. Since we started our Beauty Bible series, our winning mascaras have been Beauty Steals. On page 131, you'll find the verdicts on waterproof mascaras, but here are our testers' choices for everyday use.

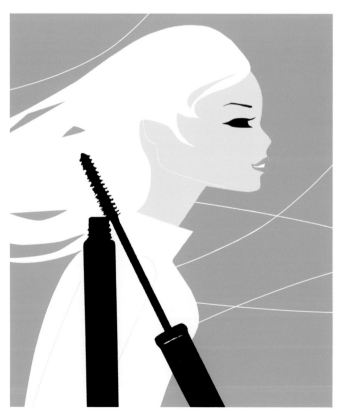

Maybelline Define-A-Lash

8.33/10 The original Maybelline mascara was created by a man called T L Williams for his sister Mabel – out of coal dust and petroleum jelly. Happily, their mascara technology has advanced apace since. This 'defining' mascara promises 'zero clumps' down to a flexible rubber wand and a lightweight formula. Two shades: Brownish Black and Black (which our testers received). Three testers gave it ten out of ten.

Testers say: 'Fell in love with this – and I am usually a Boots No 7 girl! It made my lashes long and the wand was really easy to use – an excellent product: my girlfriends asked what I was using, so it obviously made a visible difference. I am a total fan' • 'great brush, which separated as

we love

I went along; gave a natural look, which is what I wanted; with more coats, it was more thickening; made them look quite glossy, longer and quite fluttery – it didn't smudge, and I never find mascara that doesn't smudge. A great mascara' • 'economical, no irritation – and fabulous results! I have already bought another'.

Until Maybelline launched Define-A-Lash, Jo was always a devoted Lancôme Définicils girl – and then she switched. (Which tells you all you need to know…) Sarah uses Palladio Herbal Lengthening Mascara, a 'more natural' product with lots of natural waxes to condition – and it doesn't end up on her cheeks.

Max Factor False Lash Effect

Max Factor claim the stubby-handled brush 'wraps each lash right to the tip for a false lash effect', with its patented Liquid Lash™ formula. It's the favourite mascara of Marigay McKee, Harrods' director of beauty, who – when presenting a prize for this at the 2009 Cosmetic Executive Women Awards – announced that she thought they should sell it in Harrods! Just over our tenner mark, but it rivals others twice the price – and more.

Testers say: 'Applied slowly and carefully, it didn't clump at all; makes my lashes look slightly longer and thicker: I like this a lot; the length of the wand and the actual brush is excellent – I have the most miserable lashes in England and it really made a

difference' • 'Flake? No. Crumble? No. Smudge? Only if you rub your eyes' • 'lashes looked thicker and glossier' • 'very good at lengthening lashes; liked the flexible bristles – best thing is it's so longlasting; still looked fresh hours after applying and it really opened my eyes up' • 'single coat is perfect for work, but you can build it up if you want'.

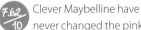

Maybelline Great Lash

Clever Maybelline have never changed the pink and green packaging of this so-distinctive mascara, which debuted in 1971 and is used by 200 million women worldwide. But it's the lash-building, conditioning formula – and the brush, with its fairly wide-spaced bristles – which opened our testers' eyes to this classic. Three shades: we trialled Very Black.

Testers say: 'Ten out of ten: goes on like a dream; no clumping; did

a great job lengthening; very natural looking; no nasty flaking, crumbling or smudging – my lashes were lovely and soft and it didn't irritate my eyes – thank you for introducing me to this wonderful mascara' • 'nice big brush made application easy; maybe a 40 per cent thickening (much better than lengthening) and it looked glossy – my 14-year-old daughter loved it and ran out to buy some!' • 'I was very excited to try this and there are great things about it: lashes are easily coated and it makes them bolder, but not in an overbearing way – the mascara is easily removed, too'.

L'Oréal Paris Volume Collagene

The key ingredient in this is volumising 'Hydra-Collagen'. The brush is huge, for quick, even application, and it comes in Black only. L'Oréal have hundreds of scientists, and the technology and design (including mascara innovations) that feature in upscale brands often trickle down to the high street later on.

Testers say: 'Excellent: a lovely product to use and really made my lashes look thicker and longer – though they're not, nowadays! Also easy to remove with my usual eye make-up remover' • 'looked longer, a little thicker and curled up at the ends' • 'absolutely no clumping; very good at lengthening and thickening; glossy, lustrous finish; no flaking or smudging' • 'a pleasure to use, mainly thanks to the excellent brush: twirling it through lashes gave excellent cover, volume, length and very good curl'.

Max Factor Masterpiece Max

7.37/10 The original Masterpiece mascara took the world by storm. This new version boasts an innovative 'Volume iFX' brush, made of flexible rubber, so the formulation transfers more easily to lashes without clumping. It contains 'heat-, abrasion- and water-resistant polymers', to last all day without smudging or smearing. Three shades (with Black for our testers).

Testers say: 'My lashes look amazing, long and thick, glossy and full – one coat looked natural, two made my lashes look really prominent – this mascara is fantastic; amazing lashes, with no smudging or flaking: I used to wear false lashes, but no need to with this!' • 'I love this and would recommend it' • 'I have short lashes and this lengthened them and opened my eyes up without looking artificial' • 'mascara is the one product I can't live without: I have tried lots, and this is brilliant because there's no risk of "tired panda" look. Ten out of ten for daytime, eight out of ten all round, because it doesn't really thicken' • 'my holy grail mascara, which gives glossy, perfect lashes every day – flawless product'.

L'Oréal Paris Telescopic Carbon Black

7.35/10 This is the choice if you want truly inky lashes: 'extreme black pigments' bind to the lashes to create a deeper, black finish, visibly lengthening lashes by up to 70 per cent. Like some of the other winners here, it has a flexible rubber 'comb', which needs practice, but then gives easy-glide application, and no clumping.

Testers say: 'This was a doddle to apply, once I got the twirling action right; the least clumpy mascara ever – my lashes are fine, few and far between; this lengthened and thickened them into really glam lashes – even made it look like I possess bottom ones' • 'the applicator is the best yet – a perfect wand' • 'my lashes looked longer and more defined – more healthy, too; it wasn't an easy product to remove, but maybe that's the price to be paid for such a longlasting and bold effect' • 'made lashes longer, more separate and slightly thicker – also very black!'.

tip **We recommend replacing mascara every three months minimum, because after that they start to clump. But if yours has started to go globby, a favourite make-up artist's emergency resuscitation is to spritz the wand with an Evian mister – tap water in a plant atomiser is fine, too. (Although obviously this isn't going be successful for waterproof formulations.)**

 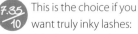

Waterproof mascaras

Finding a mascara that stays put come hell or high water (pool/rain/tears) is a big challenge. We're not going to pretend: these 'steals' performed just fine – not as well as some luxe brands we've trialled but better than many others. You could do a lot worse than these (and no, we would never have our lashes dyed – Jo had a terrible reaction from a reputable salon, and Sarah has read too many labels on hair colours that warn against putting them near your eyes).

No 7 Extreme Length Waterproof Mascara

7.67/10 Mascara success is pretty much all down to the wand design. This brush is especially 'flexible', to grip the lashes and extend them. It also allows access to hard-to-reach lashes in the corners. We dispatched Shade 01 Black.

Testers say: 'Very good at lash-lengthening, though not so hot on thickening; brush provided great separation – so no clumping; a good everyday mascara which was weepy film proof' • 'no smudges running in the rain, or the shower, and tears couldn't shift it!' • 'very natural looking, slight gloss and lashes nicely separated; loved the wand' • 'lashes looked longer and curled well' • 'rubber wand with spaced-out "spikes" so mascara went on evenly; lasted well through weepy movie; bit smudgy after a shower'.

Maybelline Define-A-Lash Waterproof

6.77/10 The non-'proofed version of this features in the previous section, with its flexible rubber wand, to help create curl, without clumping. The only shade it comes in is Very Black – but, actually, that's fine by most women we know.

Testers say: 'Went on very easily; could build up coats with no problem. Lashes look great: defined, longer, thicker – totally showerproof' • 'one of the best mascaras I have tried – and swimming-pool proof!' • 'went to my aqua aerobic class and felt a million dollars – it didn't budge; the downside is that it's hard to wash off!' • 'ten out of ten: fat lashes that last the distance!' • 'brilliant brush; so easy to separate lashes; don't clump at all: didn't run in the rain, shower, weepy movie – or when my eyes water, as they do a lot'.

Sleek MakeUP Waterproof Mascara

6.7/10 Sleek – primarily for black and Asian skins – promise this has conditioning and softening properties, is long wearing, defines eyes without clumping/smudging, yet is easy to remove.

Testers say: 'Went on very easily; no clumping, good lash lengthening and glossy finish; coped well with swimming pool, then came off easily with my usual remover' • 'good everyday mascara' • 'ten out of ten: good at lengthening, and good thickening; I would buy this' • 'brush had generous bristles, so really easy to apply; fantastic waterproofing!' • 'stayed put in a weepy movie, but didn't scare husband or dog from comforting me; easy to remove' • 'surprised at how well it performed all round, and affordable on pocket money'.

tried & tested
mineral make-up

Although it comes in powder form, mineral make-up is basically an all-in-one replacement for foundation and powder. You might be feeling a bit yada-yada-yada about it, but we do encourage you to try these winners, not least because they outperformed a few of the more costly and chi-chi mineral products found in marbled beauty halls. We are covering this category in more depth than most others because there is such a lot of interest – and not much basic information.

Prestige Skin Loving Minerals Gentle Finish Mineral Powder Foundation

7.16/10 In addition to the mineral pigments, this features a 'skin-loving mineral complex' including calcium, manganese, magnesium and potassium, plus vitamins A, C, E, shea butter and camomile extract. (We got that from the PR bumph because – after breaking a nail trying to prise the label off the bottom of the container to uncover a full ingredients list – Jo gave up.) There are eight shades, for all skin tones, including women of colour; we were sent Fair to pass on to our Beauty Bible beauty-hounds.

Testers say: 'Sometimes the powder develops a mind of its own, but if you use a little with a light hand, you avoid a messy situation! Gave a very natural finish that evened my skin tone, with sheer coverage that you could build up'•'perfect coverage on small blemishes; friends said how good my skin looked – I'm never using cream foundation again!'•'this is a godsend! My long-term acne, which meant using antibiotics and anti-inflammatory

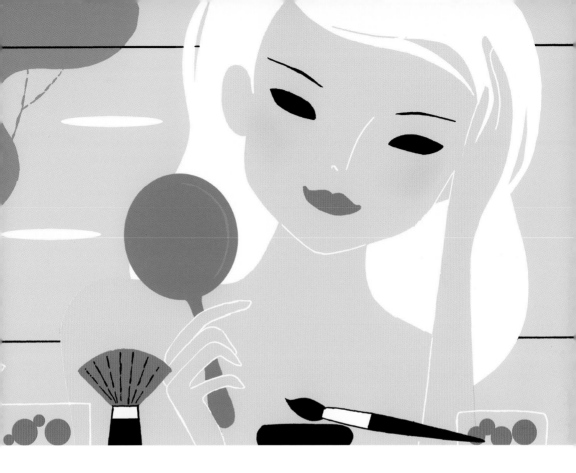

products, has cleared completely using this product; it has very light coverage and feels good on my skin' • ' would have liked instructions for mineral "virgins'" • 'much better coverage than my usual liquid foundation: I am a convert! But this is not one for your make-up bag, as the packaging isn't sturdy enough' • 'gave a more sheer natural coverage than my usual creamy foundation' • 'I was surprised that it covered light thread veins and open pores, and evened out blemishes, yet felt very light on my skin'.

L'Oréal Paris True Match Minerals

 There's a lot of talk about mineral make-up being 100 per cent natural mined mineral pigments – actually, it isn't always. Case in point: this powder also contains silicones and a few synthetics. (Although finding this out from the ingredients list was a challenge requiring a magnifying glass and, yes, even a mirror!) In a chunky Perspex pot, this incorporates a brush which can be dipped

tip

Mineral make-up is best used with a brush (a 'kabuki-style' stubby one, which is designed for the job, or a powder or blush brush does fine – though some pricier brands come with an inbuilt powder-dispensing brush). Knock off the excess, then swirl into the skin in little round movements to gradually build coverage (and you just keep going, till all your imperfections are disguised). Once you've done your basic coverage, mineral make-up guru Susan Posnick showed us a clever trick to conceal specific flaws – say, a broken vein – without having to add more coverage to the whole face. Simply dip your clean fingertip in the mineral powder, and press on to the skin, patting until it's blended.

in the product to apply, using small, circular motions; we recommend tipping a little of the powder out into a dish, then re-attaching the brush to the pot, otherwise it's a little unwieldy. It comes in six shades, which should blend with any skin tone from fair to dark (our testers had Nude Beige). It busts through our price 'ceiling' (and then a bit), but L'Oréal Paris is such a 'mass' brand that we really had to include this (and see 'We love', *opposite*, too). Some very high marks for this, with the odd low score (for messiness, not quality) that reduced the average.

Testers say: 'This is lovely. So easy to apply: almost foolproof. The only time I might wear

liquid now is if I needed a really formal "made-up" look; my 22-year-old daughter borrowed one pot and I never saw it again; an excellent everyday foundation at a sensible price' • 'surprisingly unmessy, applied with its own brush (though that could be a bit less scratchy): gives a lovely, natural, slightly matt finish, but not powdery' • 'compared with other brands, this is extremely good value' • 'not messy, but still probably better to apply before dressing, especially in black!' • 'good coverage, but didn't feel like I was wearing any foundation at all' • 'very neat packaging – spill proof, when closed, so you can carry it anywhere; the finish initially looks powdery, then

seems to react with the warmth of the skin and goes matt but not dusty, giving an overall natural effect, with even skintone, and redness covered' • 'despite being a powder, it doesn't gather in fine lines and wrinkles: seems to glide over them and disguise them; certainly did a good job disguising my open pores – I was impressed' • 'the built-in brush didn't work for me, but I did well with my Beauty Blender sponge; coverage was lovely – heavy enough to cover any blemishes, yet looked as if I was only wearing a sheer product. This is one of the lowest-priced mineral make-up products I have used and gives just about the best finish'.

Something slightly different

How to categorise this rather defeated us. Yes, it's mineral, and e.l.f. submitted it for the mineral make-up category, but, in fact, it turns out it's a complexion-boosting 'finisher' in loose powder form, which some testers liked a lot.

e.l.f. Mineral Booster

6.25/10 Super-affordable, this is a simple pot of minerals blended with cornstarch (and no chemicals), plus vitamins A, B and E and zinc. The makers, e.l.f., say 'this melts into the skin, promoting healthier skin that's noticeably silkier and smoother – gently absorbing oil and minimising the appearance of wrinkles, fine lines and pores'. It comes in just one shade – 'Sheer' – for all skintones, and is designed to be used as a complexion-boosting 'finisher'. Use it either alone (you need pretty good skin for this) or buffed over concealer and foundation (they say their own mineral products – but we think it would work over liquid, too) for extra staying power and a 'stunning porcelain matt look that will last all day'. There are two sizes; the small one is a useful trial (though the pot is too small to get most brushes into, according to testers).

Testers say: 'Top marks for this; it gave a sheer, dewy, natural coverage that was fine on its own, or over a concealer for more serious blemishes – brilliant!' • 'light, sheer coverage that settled to a soft, natural finish after a few minutes; helped cover open pores and small blemishes, though still best over a concealer for me, or a light foundation; gave a peachy finish to my skin' • 'I didn't think this product was that special until I went back to my normal powder, which looked much less natural and heavier – then I got the point!' • 'covered open pores well'.

♡ we love

Jo picked up a pot of the L'Oréal Paris True Match Minerals, *opposite*, in the States (after her make-up bag was lost in transit!) and was pretty impressed – but discovered one of the downsides of these drugstore brands, first hand: it's easy to pick up the wrong shade, as there don't tend to be any testers. Her initial choice was too pale and ashy; these mineral make-ups seem to come up slightly lighter than the shade that appears in the pot.
Sarah, too, is impressed by mineral foundations; obviously they don't give quite as dewy a finish as some liquid bases but nor do they look powdery/cakey – and using the simple application tips, *opposite*, they will cover most blemishes.

tried & tested
day creams

There are no bells and whistles on these creams (which translates as: no SPFs, whizzy anti-ageing ingredients or 'designer' jars). They're just basic creams to leave skin moisturised and comfy, day after day. Perfectly good performances, here, for some perfectly good creams. OK, so they lagged behind some of their much pricier rivals – but they left just as many trailing in their wake. Steals? For sure.

  Bioré Shine Control Moisturiser

7.12/10 One for our shiny-skinned brigade: a lightweight, oil-free moisturiser which sinks in fast. It comes in a hygienic pump action bottle, and features what Bioré call Pore Smart® Technology, with advanced oil absorbers to leave skin smooth and naturally matt. While some testers raved about it, others found it was not hydrating enough, however.

Testers say: 'Made my skin stay matt for longer, which I noticed also when I wasn't wearing make-up; I would recommend it;

it dried so quickly I could apply my make-up just a few minutes later; however much I put on it, didn't make my skin greasy' • 'skin felt velvety after application; smells fresh and pleasant, like cucumber; make-up goes on fine over it' • 'felt very fresh and cool' • 'I liked the texture initially but some days it felt a bit drying' • 'nice light texture that might suit a teenage girl' • 'I like the lightweight texture, which sinks into my oily skin almost instantly; I never use a moisturiser normally, but this made a good base, without aggravating skin'.

Weleda Wild Rose Day Cream

7/10 One thing we have divined in our years of testing is that anything with a rose scent pushes buttons with our testers. That's not the only reason they liked this all-natural, quickly absorbed cream (with oils of musk rose, peach kernel and almond, to nourish and revitalise) – but the essential-oil-derived fragrance certainly enhanced the cream's pleasure quotient. We love it ourselves, as we explain above.

Testers say: 'Very moisturising; lovely to smooth on to face, and felt it was quite calming on my red areas; lovely rosy smell, but not old fashioned; rich, creamy texture: I loved it!' • 'I had fewer blemishes when testing this product' • 'light and quickly absorbed; nice texture; skin was soft and looked smoother, not shiny' • 'my skin looked a little plumper and more even toned; flaky nose went, and make-up applied easily; lovely, velvety-soft texture that melts into the skin,

we love

leaving it very soft and dewy; also made a very effective neck cream'•'value for money; I think this is a great buy – the moisturisation is as good as more expensive products'•'my skin drank this up, more than any moisturiser I have ever used; it kept my skin moisturised during the very cold weather'•'skin is soft, supple, hydrated and looks "fresher" – I enjoyed using this and it performed well'.

 Skin Therapy Moisturising Day Cream

 This Sainsbury's range offers extraordinary value: attractive but simple packaging, and pleasing textures,

> For a good, basic, multi-tasking day cream we would both go for the Weleda range: incredibly high-quality creams for the price, formulated with entirely natural ingredients that don't cause problems for our sensitive skins. We love the Rose cream testers liked, soft-scented Iris Day Cream and good old multi-tasking Skin Food, featured on page 145.

with a raft of skin-caring ingredients including (here) vitamins and Co-enzyme Q10, in a sinks-in-fast cream. (One tester had a sensitivity reaction.)

Testers say: 'Velvety-light cream that was easily absorbed; my skin definitely looks better'•'smells very pleasant, but light'•'skin smooth and soft to touch'•' I'd say it does enhance radiance; sinks in quickly, and make-up went on smoothly; think it does have some anti-ageing benefits – skin was smoother and more radiant'•'great as a neck cream, but was too heavy for my face' •'good moisturiser – as good as other good skin creams, and probably cheaper'.

Nivea DNAge Day Cream

 The next highest-scoring product in this category is nearer to 20 than ten quid – but our rationale is that the DNAge range is one of Nivea's highest-tech creations yet, and

so it's more than 'just' a day cream. Folic acid and creatine are said to speed up cell renewal and boost vitality, while giving skin a good moisturising drink. There's an SPF15 'light filter' system (as they put it), so this could equally well have slotted into the SPF15 Moisturiser category, too.

Testers say: 'Skin was immediately soft and smooth after applying; lovely fresh smell, with luxurious feel; not at all greasy'•'very impressed with this: I didn't look ten years younger immediately, but my skin tone certainly improved'•'light cream, easy to apply and sinks in easily and quickly'•'gave lovely base for make-up'•'would buy this again and am interested in the whole range; I'm very surprised, as I've never had great experiences with Nivea before'•'my skin felt a lot softer and looked in better condition after just 24 hours'•'I've used it religiously and have become quite a fan'.

tip

'If you don't have time to wait 15 minutes between applying moisturiser and foundation, dry your face with a hairdryer on a cool setting. One of my patients told me she did this because she was tired of waiting.' *Dermatologist Dr Frederic Brandt*

tried & tested
night creams

What we look for in a night cream is simply something to make skin feel comfortable and enhance the effects of sleep, so we wake up that bit more radiant. Those featured here scored well, even beating some 'cult' creams and some luxe ones. (For true 'miracle' creams, turn to page 12.)

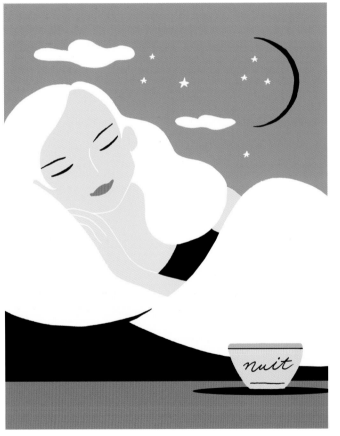

nuit

Weleda Wild Rose Night Cream ❁ ❁

8.25/10 Weleda buys more than 400 million roses a year, largely from an organic Fairtrade project in Turkey, and some make their way into this winning cream – alongside evening primrose, *Sedum purpureum* and myrrh, to protect against loss of vitality.

Testers say: 'My skin was soft, smooth and looked good, despite me being worn out' • 'smells of roses; a pleasure to put on' • 'my skin looked radiant in the morning' • 'skin looked lovely, smoother – brilliant' • 'rich, but sinks in easily' • 'skin revitalised, and pores less noticeable'.

Healthspan Nurture Intensive Night Repair Cream

7.44/10 This night cream promises to help boost skin's natural collagen levels, and reduce the appearance of fine

lines, wrinkles and age spots. Its secret is retinol, a powerful anti-ageing ingredient found in much more expensive creams. Healthspan Nurture keep prices down by direct selling.
Testers say: 'Made me look younger: husband commented I looked "particularly nice" the first evening I had it on' • 'created a temporary tightening and freshening of small lines' • 'has an instant plumping effect; I used it as a pre-make-up primer before a night out' • 'skin was moisturised perfectly without shine' • 'skin felt smoother and more even, glowing and rejuvenated, large pores seemed smaller – never had such dramatic results'.

No. 7 Protect & Perfect Night Cream

7.2/10 This creation contains a skin-firming complex with lipo-peptides to boost elasticity, radiance and moisturisation, and is meant to be used with the No. 7 Protect & Perfect Beauty Serum. It busts through our price ceiling – but per millilitre isn't much more expensive than Weleda or Healthspan Nurture. (Two testers had sensitivity reactions.)
Testers say: 'My skin feels very smooth and velvety; I loved the clean fresh smell and it did its job well' • 'skin looked smooth, almost toned, though I didn't think it was moisturising enough' • 'leaves skin feeling velvety' • 'light and silky; sinks in beautifully'.

we love

OK. Jo's completely and utterly devoted to Liz Earle Superskin Moisturiser and would probably mortgage her soul to continue to use that at night. But, like Sarah, she would happily use the Weleda Wild Rose Night Cream (opposite) if she had to.

Skin Therapy Intensive Night Recovery Cream

7.2/10 Same score as the No. 7 product, but a third of the price. Find it at Sainsbury's. This contains a 'Skin Recovery Complex' with pro-retinol, plus moisture-boosting ceramides. After four weeks, 75 per cent of testers in an independent trial felt the cream boosted radiance and firmed their skin – here's what our panellists have to add...
Testers say: 'The texture was so rich and luxurious, it glided on the skin and was absorbed almost immediately. My skin looked plumper and hydrated; much better than my usual night cream' • 'skin felt softer and firmer – this cream smells divine' • 'a colleague said I looked glowing with health' • 'a great product with fantastic results'.

Yes to Carrots C Through The Night – Night Moisturising Cream ❀

6.3/10 Yes to Carrots are all over this book, having come (almost) from nowhere to become one of the top affordable (and natural) skincare brands. This lags a little behind the others in this category, but in its fairly rich formulation you'll find veg-derived vitamins, Dead Sea minerals and ginkgo biloba for a glow by morning. One person had a sensitivity reaction.
Testers say: 'Skin noticeably more hydrated and smooth after the first night; really glowing in the morning; plumped and very comfortable; lovely texture; moisturised well and deeply; left a silky to matt finish on the skin, which looks better and younger' • 'just as moisturising as my usual night cream, but cheaper' • 'top marks: it just melts into my skin, which is now so moisturised it looks radiant, feels softer and has been less temperamental – I am now addicted!'.

double-duty
beauty

Stuck in the deep countryside without hair-styling products, we once used an anti-cellulite lotion. And guess what? It worked fine, thus proving that the basis of many products is the same. Make-up-wise, you can double or even triple up on masses of products, too. In fact, savvy beauty companies are beating the credit crunch by producing multi-taskers now. So you can use their expertise as well. Just be creative – and let us know what works for you at www.beautybible.com

tip

A good, clear, slightly gungy balm or salve (or Vaseline, if you don't mind a petroleum byproduct) is fab as a base which you can mix almost anything into. Balm is possibly the greatest multi-purpose product ever: use it for glossing lips, taming frizzies, overnight line softener, cuticle conditioner, moisturiser (face, elbows, knees, feet), even as a make-up remover.

Bronzing powder for eyeshadow: try products in any bronzing palette, mixed with balm as a lippy, as blusher (perhaps with a tad of pink), under brows… Also add along, and just under, the jawline for a more sculpted shape.

Eyeshadow pencil for brow liner: taupey colours are best; avoid anything with red in it.

Brown mascara for brow thickener: this tip comes from beauty legend Marcia Kilgore.

Glitter powder for anywhere highlighter: one high-street company is marketing its eye glitter dust (under £3) as a multi-tasker: use dry or wet on the eye, mix with lip balm for a glittery sheen, sweep pale shades on cheekbones for instant highlighter; swish across shoulders and collarbones for bare-shouldered glam. Actually, highlighters are multi-purpose, full stop – and there are lots in budget ranges.

Ivory-coloured cream eyeshadow for under-eye concealer: dot on very sparingly, then smooth a tad of your own skin-matching foundation on top.

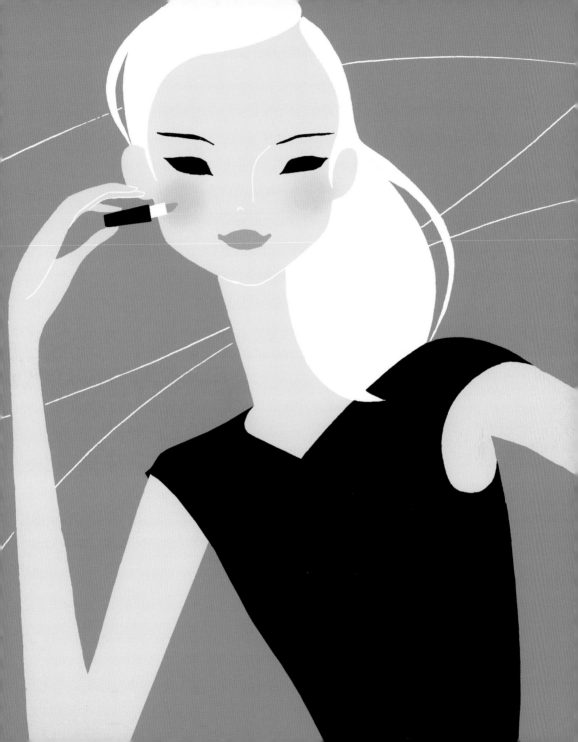

Eye make-up base as blemish concealer: do as previous page.

Rosy lipstick for blusher: a soft rosy-brown lippy looks great on cheeks; in warmer weather, try gloss for a gorgeous shimmery look. There are also specific lip 'n' cheek stain products.

Lip barrier for temp tattoo fixer: use lip fixers on brows or, for example, use the classic Lipcote lipstick sealant over temporary glitter tattoos.

Mascara for root growth: you need the right hue for your hair.

Face cream for neck cream! As make-up artist Laura Mercier says: 'The skin on your neck is basically the same as the skin on your face and hands…'

tip

Put a little baking soda in your facial cleanser to convert it into a very gentle scrub; then you can mix some more into your toothpaste to brighten and whiten your pearlies!

SPF15 moisturiser for hand cream: give your hands the same protection as your face.

Lemon juice for hair lightener and natural deo: rinse your hair in water with the juice of half a lemon and let it dry in the sun, stroke a quarter over your pits, and squeeze the rest into a glass of water to drink. Genius!

Hair styling gel for brow fixer: apply a tiny bit with ring or little finger to keep brows groomed.

Retinol face products for craggy elbow/heel treatment: it's skin, *n'est-ce pas*? So the results will be the same…

Shampoo for body wash: and vice versa!

Almond oil for bath oil, on skin, as hair conditioner: another brilliant multi-purpose product, which is all natural. PS: all body oils – eg, massage blends – make brilliant bath oils; you can always dilute them with a base oil (almond, jojoba, peach kernel, etc) if you want to make them go further. And you can rub a teensy bit on the ends of your hair to tame and gloss.

new tricks

Brands have caught on to this trend and are coming up with all sorts of useful ideas (and some which are just plain silly). Lip glosses incorporate plumping agents for a bee-sting pout. Others, sensibly, have SPF15 sunscreens. MeMeMe Ultra Duo Lipstick has colour one side and shimmer gloss the other (but the usefulness would depend on wearing down each side equally – which is probably dodgy). Cleansers and facial wipes contain exfoliating beads – but do check they are soft and rounded or you'll end up Day-Glo pink. (And you could just rub gently with a face cloth and your usual cleanser.) d:fi Extreme Shape is a nifty styling product which, used at close range, creates a mousse to prime the hair pre-heat and styling, or, held at a bit of a distance, releases high-hold hair spray for a finishing spritz.

tried & tested
multi-purpose balms

These belong in every budget-conscious beauty's life, because a single pot performs so many different tasks, from cleansing (at a pinch) to smoothing cuticles, softening lips, repairing cracked heels – you name it, basically. There are several good contenders, some of them entirely natural – and two of the top products here have also earned a place in our book, *The Green Beauty Bible*.

finger heat melts it into little slick of oil; no unpleasant residue on fingers'•'kept lips nice and soft, cleared up little dry patch on my hand, great on rough skin on feet: I'm addicted, and so are my friends'•'goes everywhere with me; problem is it's so lovely you just want to keep putting on more! Smells of lavender and tastes the same'.

Champneys Moisture Miracle Rescue Balm

8.05/10 The products in this Champneys range were created with input from real-life Champneys spa therapists, so it's never surprised us that there are so many high-performing products in the range. This is probably the most inexpensive of the lot: a little pot of TLC with a 100 per cent natural ingredient list: carnauba and beeswax, sweet almond oil and cocoa butter, with an aromatherapeutic fusion of geranium, camomile and lavender to soothe the senses.

Testers say: 'Liked the small pot, perfect for bag – works well at softening cuticles, and on dry knuckles, elbows and knees; quite a strong herbal smell'• 'softening effect really lasted, left slight residue which felt like moisture film protecting the area I applied it to; not sticky at all; quite oily and slippy, so it "travelled" well and a little went a long way'• 'solid in its pot but

Essential Care Calendula Balm
❀ ❀ ❀

7.95/10 This 100 per cent organic, totally natural pot of wonder gets its healing action from calendula and camomile, in a lubricating base of organic coconut and extra virgin olive oil, plus shea butter. Devotees have actually reported great results using this on psoriasis, but it's more widely recommended for cracked cuticles, chapped skin on fingers, elbows, heels, etc. Essential Care is a commendable

UK-based brand founded by a mother-and-daughter team who are deeply committed to creating organic skincare, and are happy to ship worldwide, while they continue to grow their business internationally. **Testers say:** 'Nourishing on the lips and made a significant difference in this area in very harsh winter weather: this is where I received most benefit' • 'I liked this product and was happy to apply on my children's skin, which is very important to me' • 'calmed a sore lip very quickly' • 'very soothing for sore, chapped knuckles; I used it on my 12-year-old son's knees before football and it really protected them' • 'very soft balm, which melted quickly on the skin' • 'a lovely, soothing, all-purpose balm, slightly oilier in texture than I might like, but pleasingly natural and effective'.

tip

If you like a funky-chunky finish to your hair, smooth a teeny bit of one of these solid balms between the palms of your hands to warm it and skim through your hair, twisting the ends for definition. Who needs hair wax?

 Rose & Co Rose Petal Salve

 Such a pretty tin. Such a pretty smell. (And, despite the fact it's so blooming cheap, Rose & Co tell us that Paris Hilton and Kate Winslet like it.) A teensy whinge from the Beauty Bible police, however: the PR bumph makes much of

the product containing 'natural ingredients such as beeswax', but neglects to mention that, like many balms out there, its key ingredient is petroleum.

Testers say: 'Fab multi-purpose, day-to-day balm: versatile enough to tackle very dry patches like heels, and more delicate bits such as cuticles; much less greasy than Vaseline, and extra marks because it smelt so good' • 'has done a great job on my cuticles and gives nails a bit of a shine' • 'excellent on dry patches; really felt as if it was nourishing them' • 'love the traditional "Grandmother" packaging; a simple and effective beauty solution, which I kept with me – as an emergency perfume as well!' • 'loved this, and it makes a really nice gift' • 'very good for controlling unruly eyebrows' • 'made elbows look much nicer' • 'a big hit with my friends, too: when I get it out in the pub or at work, all their hands fly in for some'.

And a special mention in this category goes to...

 Vaseline Pure Petroleum Jelly

 We don't usually feature a product that's a way down the list. But good old Vaseline petroleum jelly was the

♡ we love

Jo swears by natural Badger Balms: her favourite is **Tangerine Breeze**, deliciously fragranced with tangerine, mandarin, rosehip, pink grapefruit, orange and sage, in a cute badgery tin. And Sarah loves organic **Balm Balm**, particularly in Rose Geranium, for face, hands, lips – just about anything really.

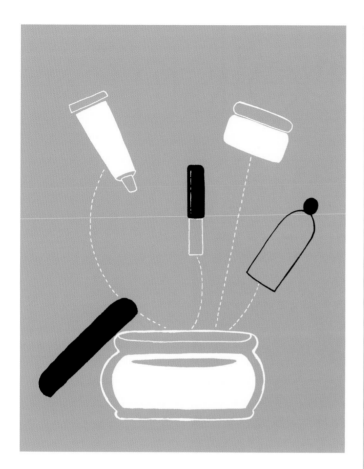

Not quite a balm, but it's brilliant!

Weleda Skin Food ❀❀

 This 'cult' product has been around since 1926, we're told! Although Weleda call it a 'balm', this multi-tasker is really a rich cream and is so useful as a moisturiser – for faces, bodies, hands, feet, elbows. It's refreshingly scented with essential oils (orange, lavender), and we also recommend it as a fabulous barrier cream in wind-chill weather.

Testers say: 'I love, love, love this product and the price means I can slap it on – it's the best face mask, kept my hands amazing through winter, softened cuticles, helped heal and protect dry patches' • 'seriously awesome on dry feet and elbows; rich, smells gorgeous and feels like it's doing good' • 'AMAZING!!! The first product ever to soothe, improve, heal and clear all my eczema and contact dermatitis.'

original 'multi-purpose' product, so we thought we'd send it to our testers – and it didn't do badly at all (except with the green babes). It's SUCH a steal – and a classic, in millions of bathroom cabinets.

Testers say: 'I love Vaseline, and despite the smell have used it since I was about 11 – it's a great "everything" balm, and provides so many beauty benefits, from lip glossing to soothing sore, dry or inflamed patches' • 'the best lip balm out – unscented, cheap and effective' • 'a great basic multi-tasker; I love to use it on grazes, too, as a protective barrier' • 'fab for cuticles, they're much less "crispy"' • 'only thing that works on my very dry, itchy lower legs, which I have scratched until they bled'.

tried & tested
nail polish

We've long believed that some inexpensive polishes can rival the offerings from luxury beauty brands, and asked our testers to trial these for both hands and feet. So: give a hand to the winning 'steal' in this category, and a bunch of others slightly further down the score stakes.

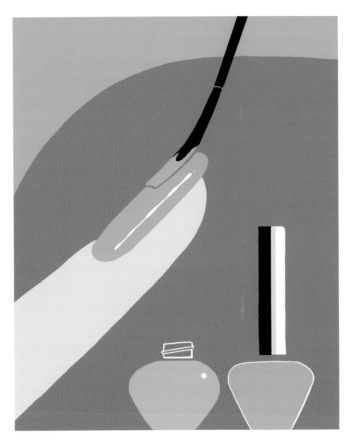

 GOSH Nail Lacquer

 Gosh, GOSH have done well in this book. The shade our testers tried in this winning polish was 044 Snow, a sort of sheer white – if you apply a single shade, the nails' own colour gives it a hint of pink. (They also do an inky black, as well as more wearable tones.)

Testers say: 'Very easy to use; nice brush shape; polish went on smoothly; I needed two coats to get a smooth effect – lasted four days before chipping' • 'touch-dry in 30 seconds – wow!' • ' good depth of shine, which did not fade until a week later' • 'looked offputting in the bottle, but very good on; made my nails look healthy and well conditioned; polish was much improved by using a base and top coat too, which also made it last longer'.

♡ *we love*

 Collection 2000 Maxiflex 5-Day Wear Polish

6.93/10 A great performance for a product from this super-affordable range, which promises five-day wear, in about 30 shades – although, to be honest, we've lost the plot as to which our testers got. Oops. We always ask for a 'wearable nude', but this was a rich, dark maroon, probably Plum Rose, or Rustique.

Testers say: 'Easy to apply; dried fast; loved the deep colour and the coverage was very even – with two coats it lasted several days' • 'two coats gave good coverage; lasted about three days without chipping on fingernails, longer on toes' • 'would work well for a night out' • 'easy to touch up • 'gave my expensive nail colours a run for their money: I bought a couple of other shades' • 'good coverage, although it didn't last long, even with two coats'.

 e.l.f. Nail Polish

6.85/10 Yet another amazing-value product from e.l.f., a quick-dry formula, with vitamin E. A couple of dozen shades: our testers had Burgundy, a deep wine colour, shot with gold.

Testers say: 'Top marks: brush gave excellent coverage, though it did shed at first; three coats needed for even colour; lasted three days without chipping; I buy high-end varnish but this is as good at a fraction of the price' • 'went on very smoothly; two coats gave a deep, even colour that I liked; dried fine, but took about ten minutes; I really liked the depth of colour and a lot of shine came through' • 'very nice colour but one coat didn't last' • 'lasted for two weeks on toenails'.

 2True Glossywear Nail Polish

6.75/10 Bargain-basement beauty brand 2True offer 36 catwalk-inspired shades. Our testers tried Shade 57 Blackberry-ish, a rich, dark hue, which they liked – although no one managed to make it last 'up to five days', as promised.

Testers say: 'Nice rich colour and quite shiny; two coats was OK, but it would probably be perfect with three' • 'I'm a beauty therapist, and while it gave fairly good coverage, the brush splays out a bit and you would need three coats to get the depth of colour' • 'nice colour and for a budget brand it did a fairly good job'.

Santé Nail Polish

6.25/10 Ah, one for the more natural nail lovers: a less-toxic-than-usual entry, from Santé: no formaldehyde, phthalates, toluene or parabens. Santé misread our instructions and submitted a rainbow of shades (they do 23, in all) which we, in turn, sent out to testers.

Testers say: 'Very practical packaging, and easy to apply; just right in terms of glossiness, too' • 'impressed with the stylish packaging' • 'went on easily over a clear base coat; I applied one coat, then a top coat and it lasted three days without chipping'.

tried & tested

nail polish remover

These are generally inexpensive, so we had lots to test. We certainly can't see a single reason ever to pay through the nose for these (unless you are a total Chanel junkie, that is: we have to say their classic bottle of pink polish remover – it looks like a downsized fragrance bottle – is adorable). Although some cheap polish removers can be incredibly drying – and smell super-toxic – those featured on these pages got very good scores. So: pay less and use generously would seem to be the nail-care mantra, here.

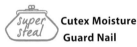 **Cutex Moisture Guard Nail Polish Remover**

 These are drenched in Cutex's Moisture Guard Formula Nail Polish Remover with Nail Whitening Formula, designed for dry, brittle nails, and the individually wrapped sachets slip neatly into a sponge bag. Although a pack of these wipes is inexpensive, using them regularly would add up. So if you like them, it would be less wasteful to use Cutex Moisture Guard remover

(Jo's top pick – see 'we love') when not travelling.

Testers say: 'Would definitely buy these: much easier; pleasant smell, everything removed, no residue; cuticles softer, nails look healthy' •

'perfect for on the go' • 'easy to remove all polish with minimum of effort' • 'not drying' • 'brilliant for travelling, because they have a foil wrapper – efficient at removing thick red polish on my toes'.

 tip

If you are ever completely stuck without polish remover, reach for some facial or body oil. It takes a bit of elbow grease and rubbing, but cotton pads, saturated with oil and held over the polish, will gradually dissolve it.

OPI Polish Remover with Aloe Vera

 This green-tinted remover features just a touch of acetone, making it a highly effective polish remover – but acetone's drying, so they've added aloe vera to counterbalance the problem. OPI recommend using this polish on either natural nails or enhancements together with their special OPI lint-free Nail Pads – although some of our testers didn't, and were still impressed.

Testers say: 'One application efficiently removed dark nail polish' • 'clear, squeezable container made it easy to get required amount' • 'my nails look better from using this: I wouldn't use any other remover now' • 'definitely recommend using with OPI Nail Pads to save on product wastage'.

 Cutex Nourishing Nail Polish Remover

 Since Cutex's main focus is nail care – and they're a legend in that world – their excellent performance in this category doesn't really come as a surprise. One of half a dozen polish-removing options, this has added vitamins and moisturising elements to condition and strengthen nails.

we love

As one of our testers says, 'Can you ever get truly excited about nail polish removers?' Hmm, perhaps not. But in general, Jo rates highly the Cutex range, which performed so well here, in particular, Cutex Moisture Guard Nail Polish Remover, since her nail problem generally is dryness. Sarah likes German brand Santé Cosmetics' organic orange nail varnish remover: it works a treat on Santé nail varnishes, though you have to work a bit harder on some other brands – mainly because it is acetate free. It's under a tenner.

Testers say: 'I left the pad on the nail for a few minutes to soak in, and it was very easy to remove polish; did seem to help strengthen my nails' • 'easy to apply and efficient, even on dark red polish; a light rubbing worked a treat; supposed to be moisturising but I just found it not overly drying' • 'polish came off straight away; no need to keep going over it; it was certainly more moisturising than a normal remover, which I find very drying, both on my nails and the surrounding skin' • 'made my nails look whiter, as promised' • 'very easy – I would buy it again'.

 Superdrug Acetone-Free Nail Polish Remover

 If we had a 'super-duper steal' category, this would be in it: you get a lot of this acetone-free blue remover for your money (it comes in a whacking 250ml bottle for a ridiculously low price). One for readers who get bored with their polish colour super-fast, we'd say.

Testers say: 'Surprisingly efficient; I only had to soak the pad twice to clean the polish off both hands' • 'smelt strong in the bottle but not on the cotton wool; in fact, for a nail varnish remover, it had quite a pleasant smell and was effective and gentle on nails' • 'a good example of a beauty necessity that doesn't have to be expensive; excellent value for money, and would last a long time. It's hard to get excited about nail polish remover but it's one of those products that can be annoying if they don't work – ie, you have to scrub your nails! Superdrug has provided a good product that does what it says, so ten out of ten for value and performance'.

tried & tested
cuticle treatments

OK, so these may be pretty low down the priority list when it comes to spending, but there were some very high individual scores. Cuticle smoothers help the many nail-obsessed women we know maintain a perfect 'ten' (nails, that is) – and, we chorus, why pay more, when there are high-performing products like these? The bonus is that, used regularly (we emphasise), these will all help strengthen nails, making them strong but flexible – the nail grail! NB: you only need a very little.

The Body Shop Almond Oil Nail & Cuticle Treatment

7.88/10 This did well, both as a cuticle smoother and as a nail treatment (see page 152), and we're not a bit surprised: Jo keeps one of these very useful pen-style nail tools in her handbag. It's a clever design: twist the top and the smoothing, almond-oil-based treatment emerges on to the brush (think YSL Touche Eclat). The genius bit, though, is a built-in rubber 'hoof-stick', which lets you push the cuticles back after massaging in the lightweight formula.

Testers say: 'I was so delighted to get this! My nails are horrible, short, and tear off when they get to any length – just wipe this on, use the hoof part, nails look very glossy – and it works! My nails are much stronger' • 'fabulous! My nails are noticeably improved; I love putting on the oil – I'm really pleased' • 'long-term improvement in my cuticles – they are softer and less ragged; very easy to carry around and use regularly' • 'nails stronger, more flexible; this made a real difference to my badly damaged post-acrylic nails'.

Burt's Bees Lemon Butter Cuticle Creme ❀

7.87/10 A little pot of softly lemon-scented magic, which melts at body temperature – based on sweet almond oil, cocoa butter, candelilla wax, rosemary extract and the signature citrus oil. Burt's Bees say that it is '94.91 per cent natural' (we like their precision!). Like The Body Shop product, *left*, this gained several 'ten's.

Testers say:: 'My flaky, weak nails looked instantly better – softer cuticles and shiny pink nails; after two weeks, they were much

tip

If you don't want a cuticle treatment, you can certainly make do with one of our multi-purpose balms, see page 143. But we have been known to smear a bit of butter on our cuticles – saves wasting what's left on the side of the plate – and it is surprisingly effective.

healthier – and this was winter'
• 'neat tin with solid balm that you could just rub in at your desk'
• 'softer cuticles, shinier nails'
• 'love the lemon smell'•'gives nails a nice shine and definitely made parched-looking cuticles supple and healthier instantly'
• 'love the retro packaging'.

Mavala Soothing Shea Butter Cuticle Care

6.60/10 Nail-nourishing minerals feature in this rich cream, softening and 'feeding' the cuticle to make for easier removal. (And Mavala, of course, are legendary in the nail world

for everything from polishes to hand creams.)

Testers say: 'Ten out of ten for this very rich cream – a little goes a long way – definitely improves the look of nails and cuticles, particularly with continued use'
• 'cuticles softer and nails shiny and stronger after two weeks' use'
• 'very practical small tube; nice thick cream with an almost minty smell'•'noticeable improvement in cuticles; hands looked more "groomed"'•'my hands are my age giveaway but this conditioned cuticles, making them less raggedy, and nails more glossy'.

 Badger Soothing Shea Butter Cuticle Care ❀ ❀

6.50/10 We're fond of the Badger brand, which seems to have a little tin of all-natural goodness for most

beauty challenges. This balm (which melts on contact) contains shea butter and sea buckthorn berry extract for cuticle TLC, softly scented with essential oils of rose geranium, ginger, cardamom, rosemary, mandarin and lemongrass.

Testers say: 'Top marks; after redecorating, my nails were very dry and damaged, short and splitting, ridged and very unattractive – immediately after using this my cuticles were less visible, nails looked buffed, and the ridges less noticeable; after two weeks, nails growing – and more flexible – cuticles soft, and I'm no longer embarrassed by them!'•'good on top of polish; looked like a topcoat'•'also used to moisturise my very dry hands and as a soothing lip balm'•'love this product: it works, and is ideal to carry in your handbag'.

 we love

Jo carries The Body Shop 'hoof-stick' product (see opposite) with her, but at night adds a simple dab of inexpensive sweet almond oil on to each nail, and massages it into her cuticles. We reckon a bottle could last several years, and you don't get much more of a 'steal' than that. Sarah massages in any oil she can find – and manicurists say, despite her 'country' nails, her cuticles are always in good condition.

tried & tested
nail treatments

Ideally, nails should be flexible but strong, so they don't snap when challenged by peeling off sticky labels, getting those beastly bits of plastic off jars and bottles, gardening, etc. There are lots of expensive nail-strengtheners out there – but the selection featured here put in a strong performance, ensuring that neither the bank nor your nails should be broken. As with all such products, however, you have to use them 24/7 – they don't work sitting on the bathroom shelf – and they may take some time, as nails grow very slowly.

Perfect 10 Super Strength

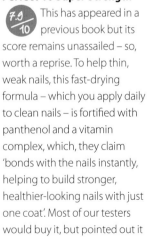

7.9/10 This has appeared in a previous book but its score remains unassailed – so, worth a reprise. To help thin, weak nails, this fast-drying formula – which you apply daily to clean nails – is fortified with panthenol and a vitamin complex, which, they claim 'bonds with the nails instantly, helping to build stronger, healthier-looking nails with just one coat'. Most of our testers would buy it, but pointed out it only worked while it was on – ie, it's a temporary effect.

Testers say: 'The strength when applied was phenomenal and the shine was divine, but when I took it off, my nails were no better' • 'gives an acrylic-like coating; made my nails feel stronger and they appeared to grow while I used it; fine, as long as I was using the product' • 'easy to apply to my weak, flaky, peeling nails, which become stronger and more flexible' • 'great staying power'.

The Body Shop Almond Oil Nail & Cuticle Treatment

7.88/10 We asked our testers to try this both as a cuticle treatment, short term, and over months as a nail strengthener – and it performed well on both counts. As you can read on page 150, it's based on almond oil and comes with a 'hoof stick', to keep cuticles tidy.

Testers say: 'Very simple and quick to use; after two weeks, my damaged nails look completely different – still not perfect, but far better than before' • 'nails were shiny, whiter and cleaner' • 'definitely made my terrible nails a bit better' • 'nails seem stronger and more flexible' • 'after about a month my nails were stronger and more flexible'.

Boots Original Formula Cuticle Oil

7.66/10 We love the Boots Original Formula range, for which Boots plundered their extraordinary packaging archive to come up with wonderfully nostalgic bottles and labels. The

we love

dropper-top bottle makes for easy application and looks good on the bedside table – so it's handy for use last thing at night. At the time of going to press this was a fiver – our ceiling for a SuperSteal – and it's certainly the cheapest product on this page.

Testers say: 'Magic! I have never used anything which has given such quick, good and longlasting results; my nails are very flexible, look strong and healthy – friends compliment me on them!' • 'great product; my nails are becoming stronger and less liable to break; they've grown really long' • 'loved the vintage-looking box – really pretty – and the dropper is easy to use; I've only had one broken nail – better than usual' • 'nails felt less brittle; practical packaging, and loved the rose smell'.

Champneys Nail & Cuticle Wonder Oil

 The natural ingredients in this 'spa manicure formula' include richly nourishing sweet almond, rice germ and meadowfoam seed oil, providing 'intensive care' for brittle nails. It has a plastic built-in angled stick in the lid, to help dab on to nails.

Testers say: 'Top marks; my nails were very brittle, short and prone

---

To boost her nails, Jo returns time and again to a simple bottle of apricot kernel oil – which is rich in A, B and E vitamins, and wonderfully nail nourishing (see DIRECTORY for sources). The pricier Essie and Cowshed products she likes to use are both based on apricot oil – but a basic bottle of the oil itself is the more-dash-than-cash option, as *Vogue* would say. Sarah's nails are adversely affected by her horses – and are officially the despair of manicurists. Meanwhile, one tip – never let anyone buff weak nails to make them smooth for polish: it leads to weaker ones.

---

to breaking; after two months, they were more flexible and didn't break as easily – am impressed' • 'my nails have more sheen and look healthy; I have fewer hang nails' • 'a manicurist told me the nails on the "treated" hand were stronger and in better condition than the other hand' • 'I actually loved this and the smell; it made my nails stronger over two months' • 'very good applicator' • 'I wouldn't normally consider this sort of product but after trying on one hand I can clearly see the benefits – I love it'.

Crabtree & Evelyn La Source Intensive Nail & Cuticle Therapy

 The La Source range is one of Crabtree & Evelyn's bestsellers, with its

---

fresh blue packaging and equally fresh fragrances. This small, nozzled tube makes for easy smoothing into nails of the strengthening elements, which include panthenol and keratin (a protective protein found in nails and hair).

Testers say: 'I've never had a manicure before because I was so embarrassed about my nails, but after using this for a couple of months I had my first one three weeks ago!' • 'my brittle nails have definitely improved and are stronger, and they look a lot neater' • 'my dry nails are a bit more flexible and stronger – certainly longer and not breaking; a manicurist also noticed the improvements' • 'you only need a tiny blob, so it's very cost effective' • 'great alternative to a nail oil; lovely-to-use cream'.

tried & tested
pressed powder

We all want to shine – but in a good way. So, these pressed powder bargains are handbag must-haves for those with a tendency to gleam as the day wears on. (Though, as an alternative, we've also included the only affordable shine-blotting tissues that impressed our testers, *overleaf*.)

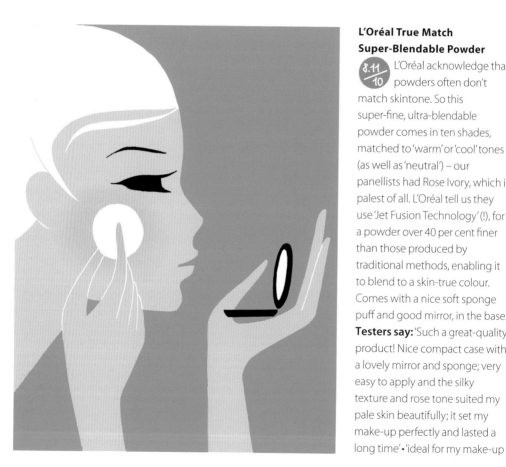

L'Oréal True Match Super-Blendable Powder

8.11/10 L'Oréal acknowledge that powders often don't match skintone. So this super-fine, ultra-blendable powder comes in ten shades, matched to 'warm' or 'cool' tones (as well as 'neutral') – our panellists had Rose Ivory, which is palest of all. L'Oréal tell us they use 'Jet Fusion Technology' (!), for a powder over 40 per cent finer than those produced by traditional methods, enabling it to blend to a skin-true colour. Comes with a nice soft sponge puff and good mirror, in the base. **Testers say:** 'Such a great-quality product! Nice compact case with a lovely mirror and sponge; very easy to apply and the silky texture and rose tone suited my pale skin beautifully; it set my make-up perfectly and lasted a long time' • 'ideal for my make-up

we love

bag; I liked the overall look and it covered my oily T-zone well, and set my make-up' • 'I have melasma [pigmentation] from being on the pill for 20 years and it covered that easily; make-up lasted all day' • 'mattified, evened skin tone, toned down blemishes'.

In Jo's make-up bag you'll find No 7 Perfect Light Pressed Powder, because it's mattifying, but not 'flat' – there's a subtle luminescence to it. (Just over the tenner mark, though – so her next-best choice is Bourjois Mineral Radiance Compact Powder – the same product she chooses as a bronzer, in Hâlé, but here in English-rose pale shade, Vanille.)

Maybelline Dream Matte Powder

7.5/10 A 'jet-milled' formula gives this its 'air-soft' feel, Maybelline explain, and the fine micro-pigments offer soft and smooth application, in five shades (our testers were assigned Rose Ivory). Like the L'Oréal winner, it comes with a pull-out mirror and suede-touch puff, but after breaking two nails, Jo gave up trying to get to them.

Testers say: 'I usually have a much more expensive brand and this compares really well – such good value. Finish was very natural – good with my skintone – and kept foundation in place all day' • 'this gave great coverage, despite six hours of wear and tear' • 'extremely useful compact, fits into any bag; good mirror and puff; not messy to use and easy to blend in' • 'fine, silky powder that gave matt natural finish and worked well to mattify shine'.

 Super steal

Collection 2000 Shine Away Compact Powder

7.2/10 In a compact that's prettily decorated with sort of Art Nouveau-ish flowers, this offers a particularly generous mirror. As to the formula, in three shades (Light, Medium and Deep – our testers tried the first), it's said to deliver up to ten hours of wear, and contains a 'Skin Correct Complex', to minimise breakouts, with anti-bacterial and anti-inflammatory properties, also helping reduce excess oil production.

Testers say: 'Very impressed – it was easy to use, gave a matt natural finish which blended with my skintone, and lasted for the promised ten hours' • 'reduced shine and gave good natural-looking finish' • 'fine, silky texture; evened out red patches on my cheeks and chin' • 'easily as good as my fairly expensive brand, for a lot less money'.

 Super steal

17 Pressed Powder

6.88/10 A simple, silky-smooth powder from Boots that is dermatologically tested and fragrance-free. In three shades (Neutral was in our testers' packages). The compact is exactly the same as Collection 2000, with the generous mirror – but no flowers on the outside and no sponge.

Testers say: 'Gave a great finish over liquid foundation; long-lasting with only the occasional touch-up required after being out in the elements' • 'I tried it with my own make-up sponge and a foundation brush, and liked the brush look best' • 'very easy to blend with my own brush, and a perfectly adequate mirror; gently balanced my skintone and set my make-up' • 'a great product if you use just the right amount; if you brush on one sweep too many, it goes chalky and you look about 15 years older!' • 'a bargain'.

tried & tested
loose powder

Nothing is better for 'setting' make-up than loose powder – and keeping shiny and/or oily areas matt. But can a 'steal' rival the pricier options out there? Having tested lots, we can put our hands on our hearts and say: these are shining stars, at great prices. (Or, rather, 'un-shining' stars.) Please do remember, though, that these are intended to grace your dressing table, not to be transported round in your handbag – for on-the-go touch-ups, a pressed powder compact is the thing, so turn to page 154 for the winners in that category.

 Make-up by Barbara Daly

Super-Sheer Loose Face Powder

6.96/10 This powder is ultra-fine, almost weightless – and translucent, of course, so it works on all skin tones. And boy, do you get a bang for your buck from Barbara's range: this is a dinky, chunky, square compact which features a good mirror in the lid and a down-sized powder puff, for application on the run. Barbara's own tip for this: 'If you have applied too much blusher, apply a little powder using the puff. This will help soften the colour and blend it into the skin.'

Testers say: 'A great buy for a supermarket product; compares very favourably with much more expensive products' • 'fine, silky, light, airy texture, which balanced skintone and gave a natural finish; certainly set my make-up' • 'really like the neat, clever design' • 'worked well on shine and didn't need to reapply on my oily T-zone' • 'gave a natural finish and

Corn Silk Translucent Loose Face Powder

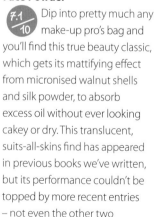

7.1/10 Dip into pretty much any make-up pro's bag and you'll find this true beauty classic, which gets its mattifying effect from micronised walnut shells and silk powder, to absorb excess oil without ever looking cakey or dry. This translucent, suits-all-skins find has appeared in previous books we've written, but its performance couldn't be topped by more recent entries – not even the other two

creditable performers, below. So we've elevated it to the 'Beauty Bible Hall of Fame', where this award-winner belongs.

Testers say: 'Helped to balance my skintone, even when I wasn't wearing foundation' • 'silky smooth – this product is a brilliant find; I was really impressed' • 'very natural finish with a tiny sparkle – very pretty' • 'the black and gold packaging makes you feel as though you've raided your mother's make-up bag'.

balanced my skintone well; my make-up lasted much longer than without it – a real bargain'.

Collection 2000 Perfecting Minerals

6.44/10 We probably should have trialled this in the mineral make-up category, but when you're sending out 2,300 different products… Well, this got dispatched to ten testers who tried it as a basic loose powder. And then, we're thinking: why not? A lot of mineral make-up powders would probably perform well simply as a face powder. Our testers really liked it – so why not have a try yourself? This one comes in three shades (our testers trialled No 3 Natural Beige), complete with a generous flat brush (some testers reported this was a moulter!). The sieve in the lid to dispense the powder has quite large holes, so be sure you're not overdoing it.

tip

For a truly seamless finish, Laura Mercier's UK make-up genius Trevor O'Keefe says you should pick up loose powder with your brush (from the lid), then swirl on the back of your hand to distribute the powder evenly among the bristles before putting them to your face.

Testers say: 'Very fine, soft texture; lovely to apply; really liked the natural subtle finish; it evened skintone and I was shine-free all day' • 'absorbed shine but didn't make my face look "flat"; lasted well on oily areas' • 'I use powder to set make-up and this gave a soft, subtle finish: not cakey' • 'gave sheer cover, which is what I like; didn't look like I had anything on'.

As an alternative for quick 'un-shines', try using a blotter!

The Body Shop Natural Powder Facial Blotting Tissues

 Adding a whisk of powder is the fastest way to blot shine – but if you do it too often, it can lead to caking. Another option is to use a shine-blotting sheet, which 'lifts' oil off the face: this little packet of shine defiance contains 65 sheets, and though they're impregnated with powder, they won't ever cake – simply blot over make-up for mattness on demand.

Testers say: 'Ten out of ten for my summer shiny complexion; I used this rather than reapply powder – stopped the shine quite well, and almost made my make-up look freshly applied. Brilliant' • 'I forgot my powder compact when I stayed at a friend's and used these instead – they did exactly the same job and my skin looked lovely!' • 'left my skin silky, smooth and matt' • 'so easy to use'.

we love

Shine isn't really Jo's problem, but she just loves the way that the Barbara Daly make-up – featured here – allows for very targeted application with the almost dolly-sized puff, so it's become a staple in her at-home kit. Sarah occasionally uses a mineral powder to set make-up for evenings out – so Collection 2000 Perfecting Minerals is quite alluring for her.

tried & tested
spot zappers

One of the biggest beauty challenges is healing unsightly zits quickly. Our highest-ever scoring products in this category cost almost ten times more than these winners – but they performed well for the price.

Most products we trial get incredibly consistent scores, but not spot-zappers. The average scores here can't reflect the fact that some testers found a product completely nixed their blemishes – while others declared it a total flop. With so many different triggers for spots (lifestyle, stress, as well as bacterial issues) you may have to do a bit of trial and error to find the product that works best for you. But since these are all true steals, that isn't such a big drain on your purse. We asked testers to report on progress over three days, and amazingly, some reported improvement in 24 hours. NB: do follow the instructions – one tester thought a single application should perform a miracle.

 The Body Shop Tea Tree Oil Blemish Stick ❀

 This has long been a winner in this category. And since we've never found anything as cheap that's matched its score, it's definitely worthy of another starring mention. This light, translucent gel – packed with naturally antiseptic and anti-bacterial tea tree oil, plus sea algae to help prevent over-drying – comes with a sponge applicator wand. The Community Traded tea tree oil is sourced from the Bundjalung Aboriginal tribal group in Australia, who 'have known about the healing powers of tea tree for 40,000 years, give or take' so The Body Shop tell us.

Testers say: 'This product reduced redness in an aggravated spot' • 'after the spot had dried up, there was no red mark' • 'spot healed entirely in three days – I will buy this again' • 'handy to carry around' • 'kept the area clean and fresh'.

Essential Care Organic First Aid Lotion ❀ ❀ ❀

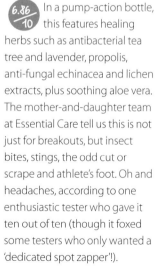 In a pump-action bottle, this features healing herbs such as antibacterial tea tree and lavender, propolis, anti-fungal echinacea and lichen extracts, plus soothing aloe vera. The mother-and-daughter team at Essential Care tell us this is not just for breakouts, but insect bites, stings, the odd cut or scrape and athlete's foot. Oh and headaches, according to one enthusiastic tester who gave it ten out of ten (though it foxed some testers who only wanted a 'dedicated spot zapper'!).

Testers say: 'Spots definitely dried up and less inflamed – by day three they were very faint; the cream had a nice clean antisepticky smell; didn't sting at all' • 'liked the calming lavender smell and the product did the job; a raw-looking spot healed well and quickly, and the red mark faded' • 'the spot only ever became slightly coloured and by day six it was invisible' • 'a very useful little tube to have around'.

 Tisserand Tea Tree Blemish Stick

 Tea tree oil is again the key antibacterial ingredient in this wand-style, handbag-friendly product, along with wild-crafted kanuka oil and astringent witch hazel.

Testers say: 'Tried on red lump spot on chin: very easy to apply; slight sting, but no tighter: it dried out the spot without drying skin around, and did speed up healing' • 'it did sting at first but I found that reassuring – spot went totally after three days. This lived up to its claims – hoorah!' • 'possibly not "industrial" enough for a big angry spot, but I felt it kept the area clean, and helped it run its course more pleasantly' • 'very impressed: white spots disappeared really quickly, red spots took longer but healed much more quickly than usual'.

tip

If you use a product with a wand-style applicator, wash it at least once a week to keep it clean and totally free from bacteria. (Yes, there are lots of antibacterials in these products, but good hygiene is so important with problem skins.) Use the same technique as for washing any brush or sponge: smoosh a mild shampoo or hand cleanser into the sponge tip and rinse well, then repeat until it's 100 per cent clean. Leave to dry thoroughly somewhere warm.

Burt's Bees Herbal Blemish Stick ❀❀

 This captures essential oils and herbal ingredients: borage seed, calendula flower and yarrow, parsley seed extract, willow bark, lemon, fennel, juniper and eucalyptus oil.

Testers say: 'I tried this on a red lump I've had for months; after

two days there was little lump left and hardly any redness; the most effective spot treatment I've used in this form' • 'didn't sting at all, dried almost instantly and did the job' • 'made a huge red hard lump less angry and nearly gone by day three' • 'a miracle blemish buster! A small red spot appeared on my cheek before Christmas: with three applications, looked better within a day; by day three there was no sign it had ever been there'.

 Free Zone Rapid Results Treatment Cream

Sainsbury's Free Zone range targets spots and blackheads with a wide choice, including this cream-formulation product. It's a good option for adolescents on a budget, as the ingredients are effective, but not as harsh and skin-stripping as many teen-targeted products.

Testers say: 'Red lump improved considerably in three days; gentle but effective; no dryness or harshness' • 'two red prominent spots disappeared in three days – great high-street find to have in an emergency' • 'would definitely buy, since this is as good as any product I've ever used for this purpose; I loved the texture being a cream, rather than a gel'.

sun tanning

Which product does what, when and for who

We are beauty editors. We know our onions. (Or rather, our moisturisers, foot files and mascaras.) Organising these Tried & Testeds is a military operation, which, in general, runs super-smoothly – and then we got to tanning products… If even we were thoroughly confused, we simply do not know how a non-beauty editor finds her way around this section of a high-street chemist or supermarket because the names don't tell you what the products do, all the packaging looks the same (all orange and gold, basically), and today, you're almost overwhelmed by choice. But, after some hard work, we really feel we can help you.

Fake (or self) tans:

Self- (aka fake) tans for face and/or body: these take a few hours to develop, and may or may not be coloured (so you can see where you've put them); they will last a few days. Some offer sun protection (which you can discount, basically, as it's only enough for a couple of hours). For faces, we prefer to use a daily/gradual tan, because it looks more natural (see next point).

Daily (aka gradual) self-tanners: these are basically a moisturiser for face and/or body, mixed with a little bit of fake tan. You apply them daily, to build up to a gradual, subtle, golden glow over five to seven days, then top them up every two to three days. They won't wash off – and, because they don't streak or patch, they are a very low-risk option for self-tan novices. We also like them better than self-tan for faces.

Leg tints: these are instant-fixes, which give you a wash-off (with soap and water, not rain), tan for the day – so they're brilliant for when your pastry pins need some instant help.

Tinted moisturisers: another instant fix, this time to give your face a gorgeous glow; some of these products also feature an SPF15 sunscreen.

Sun protection products:

SPF15 moisturisers: day creams with a sunscreen for low-risk days (every day, for us), but the sun protection won't last for a long day at the beach. Some are tinted, and we tested those, too.

Sun protection for face and/or body: these sunscreens all come in different SPFs (sun protection factors): some have a bit of colour to give you a tint as you tan. You need them to protect your skin if you are planning any concentrated time in the sun.

After-suns: moisturising and soothing preps to help prolong your tan and calm any sunburn (which you should avoid at all costs); these may also have a bit of a tan boosting colour.

We hope that makes things clearer (and will now go and lie down with a cold flannel on our heads after the stress of peering at all this packaging on your behalf).

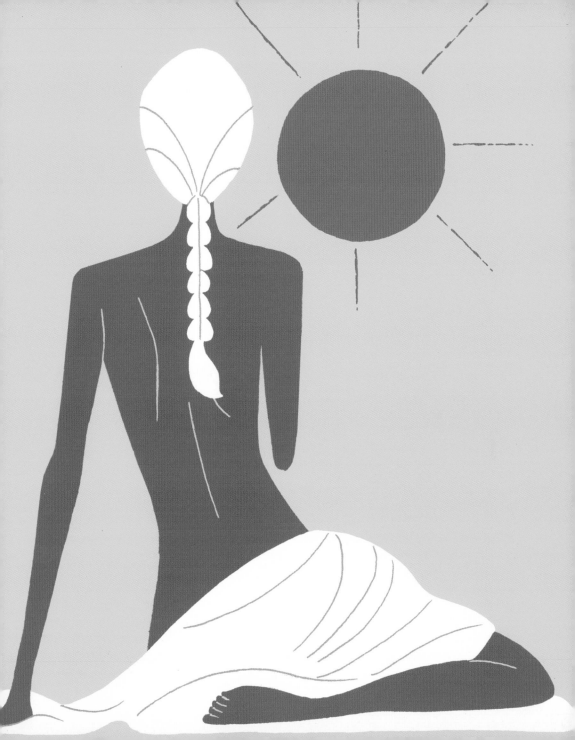

tried & tested
self-tans

We were disappointed not to have more to shout about in this category, because we certainly sent out loads to testers. To be honest, the more expensive tanners did better, but we have identified a few here that deserve gold stars – three for bodies, including two that bronzed faces, too (but do also see page 165 for a gradual facial self-tan).

Soleil Beauty Self-Tanning Spray

 7.2/10 A jolly good score for this supermarket (Tesco) own-label, self-sun product, which has what they describe as an 'easy-to-use, glide-on formula', together with an antioxidant complex. It spritzes on, which some people find makes for a more even application, though it does have to be rubbed in. Best for bodies, we think, though some testers did manage to use it on their faces successfully.

Testers say: 'Fine, untinted mist, with pleasant temporary smell, that sinks in very quickly; no tacky film; very natural colour in a few hours; works well for me' • 'took a while to get used to applying it evenly, but once I got the hang, it was easy to use and lasted well' • 'as a total tan virgin, this was quite a good experience – having a bit of colour on my pasty skin did make me feel better' • 'loved this product – much better than the one I normally use: looks like I spent a couple of days in the sun' • 'smelt surprisingly fresh on application – not like some other fake tans, which smell more like curry!'.

♡ we love

In her attempt to unravel the confusion about the Garnier Ambre Solaire No Streaks Bronzer, mentioned here, Jo tried it on herself – and was wowed with the results. She is now an occasional user (preferring generally to use wash-off tans, as a rule). Sarah's legs – often hidden under jodhpurs when's she's in the sun – are the only bit that need help, and she tends to opt for a leg tint, simply for the time factor (ie, it's usually a last-minute rescue job).

Lavera Self-Tanning Lotion ❀ ❀

 7.09/10 Good to have a new addition to the list of fake-it possibilities for natural glow-getters: this appears in our 'green book', and is suitable for use both on the body and the face. (We always suggest going 50:50 with moisturiser, the first time you try this.) From the German all-natural brand – in no-nonsense packaging – it features aloe vera, vitamin E and green tea for extra skin nourishment, and is subtly scented with rosewater, lavender flower water and essential oils.

Testers say: 'Having had breast cancer, I am wary of using fake tan on my upper body, but would very happily use this: sinks in quickly and gives a lovely, natural, very light golden colour – does need daily top-ups, though, owing to the lightness' • 'very pleasant to use; flowery smell when applied and then nothing; sinks in quickly, leaving a smooth, silky finish and pale honey colour' • 'absolutely realistic light gold; I'm now very optimistic about going bare legged in the summer; I'd have given it ten out of ten if they'd included a pair of gloves'.

Garnier Ambre Solaire No Streaks Bronzer

 6.42/10 As we've pointed out, the packaging for summer sun products can be

tip

We can't say this often enough! If you want good results, exfoliate and moisturise thoroughly before you apply a fake tan – then repeat from the day after application. Although doing this may shorten the 'lifespan' of your tan (hastening the need for re-application), it will stop your tan becoming dull and 'lacklustre'. (Avoid nut-based scrubs, though, which can lead to patchiness.) The backs of hands tend to fade fastest, so, if you notice this happening, top them up every other day with a gradual/daily self-tanner.

brain-bogglingly confusing. So, based on the blurb on the packaging – 'Medium bronze no-streaks bronzer natural dry body mist' – we were persuaded this was an instant leg tint (page 166). But, no! It's a self-tanning

spray mist, and, despite being asked leg-tint-related questions, testers came back with the following positive comments. (Jo finally figured this out after using it on herself – and was so taken with it, she now uses it – see 'we love', *opposite*). NB: this mist shouldn't need rubbing in, unlike the Tesco winner – though one tester found it did (we suspect she didn't exfoliate, and that's why it was patchy). A body product, rather than for faces.

Testers say: 'Surprisingly pleasant and easy to use; people thought it looked really natural; no giveaway rub-off marks; lifted my spirits, looking at the natural glow on my arms and legs' • 'a treat! Easy to use; no mess, rubbing it in; great for the party season, too' • 'lovely apricot fragrance' • 'dries very quickly – I needed several applications, though, on my medium skintone' • 'spray works in all directions, so it was easy to do the back of my legs; felt tacky for 10-15 minutes; developed in three hours to a lovely golden bronzy colour' • 'I needed a few sessions to practise before I was confident that I wouldn't go around looking like a tiger – but now I'd be happy to go bare legged with this'.

daily self-tanners

These daily self-tans have revolutionised the faking process, building up gradually over days. The 'original' self-tans can dry skin and you might emerge scarily dark: these give gentle tanning, while quenching skin with moisture. For a slow (and affordable) glow, look no further.

Nivea Sunkissed Skin Firming Gradual Tan Body Lotion

8/10 According to Nivea, this fresh-scented lotion contains grapeseed oil to condition skin and give it the promised 'firming' action. Our testers tried the Fair-Medium Skin version. In Nivea's in-house trials, 94 per cent said it left skin feeling supple and soft, with 87 per cent observing an even, flawless-looking tan.

Testers say: 'I liked the very subtle, realistic colour – the kind of colour my skin would go naturally' • 'enough to make me brave enough to go tightless for a special occasion' • 'consistency was just right and absorbed well' • 'doesn't streak and doesn't make you orange' • 'I would buy it again: it's no hassle, provides me with just enough colour to make me look healthy, and smells very nice – a big plus' • 'faded evenly'.

Vie At Home Summertime Skin

7.95/10 Just a bit over our £10 'ceiling', but as it scored so highly, we included it. It looks like an aerosol can, but dispenses a rich, ozonically scented milk. Some testers found one application gave a good colour, which could be topped up every two to three days; others needed the (intended) daily top-up.

Testers say: 'A dream to use: everything perfect – texture, smell, etc; easy to apply; sinks in quickly and gives skin a subtle tint immediately, then develops a deeper colour' • 'gave a pleasant pale honey colour on my fair skin, which deepens over days; nice and natural' • 'brought colour to my milk-bottle pins; didn't stain bed clothes!' • 'used over a few days, colour developed nicely: friends thought I had been away!'

tip

You can still do what we (and every other beauty editor) always used to, before this category was invented: mix your regular self-tanner half and half with facial moisturiser or body lotion. You avoid an extra bottle on the dressing table that way (and extra expense). NB: as our testers found, you need to exfoliate first – always!

Sunkiss my face

Garnier Skin Naturals Summerface 12Hr Moisturising Cream Sun-Kissed Look

 6.37/10 Basically, the slightly creamier face version of the winning apricot-scented Garnier product below. The (short-lived) smell put off some testers.

Testers say: 'My husband noticed the soft honey glow, which took two days to develop; I felt healthy and glowing' • 'took three days to see any real colour, and needed to maintain daily' • 'smelt lovely and peachy' • 'great light moisturiser, put it on – and off you go!' • 'realistic and really lifted my complexion' • 'sank in quickly and didn't feel sticky'.

Garnier Skin Naturals Summerbody Moisturising Lotion Sun-Kissed Look

6.81/10 Again with just a hint of self-tanning ingredient, this features camomile extract (for its soothing properties) and apricot, which gives a pleasant, light and subtle scent. It promises 12 hours of moisturisation.

Testers say: 'A joy to use; like a very good body lotion; smelt good enough to eat; sank in very quickly – made me feel healthy' • 'lovely, soft, natural colour but did fade in patches – maybe I should have used an exfoliant!' • 'faded evenly, but I do exfoliate' • 'applied at night, and by morning I had a subtle glow' • 'impressed with the feel, look – and fruity smell!' • 'much nicer than other fake tans I've used'.

 Neutrogena Norwegian Formula Nourishing Glow Body Moisturiser

 6.57/10 The tanners we tried seem to promise either 12-hour or round-the-clock moisturisation – this is the latter type. Two options: Normal to Fair Skin, or Normal to Dark Skin (testers trialled the former).

Testers say: 'Really good moisturiser; gave a good even colour; half-decent smell (which disappeared shortly)' • 'sank in quickly' • 'gave nice light golden colour, which got more even every day' • 'a really good self-tan moisturiser' • 'great consistency; gave an effortless natural tan; I enjoyed using it' • 'realistic look; faded evenly; great moisturising'.

L'Oréal Nutri-Summer 24 Hour Moisturising Lotion

 6.56/10 L'Oréal say this is enriched with Hydralium™ complex, to leave skin moisturised for 24 hours. We like the way that it leaves little gold particles on the skin!

Testers say: 'Straightforward to use; nice smell; great texture, like rich body lotion; natural glow' • 'pleasant flowery smell' • 'sinks in quickly; no trace on clothes at all; colour builds daily, and is even if you apply it carefully' • 'perfect self-tanner for my fair, freckly skin'.

Dove Summer Glow Beauty Body Lotion

6.25/10 This lotion comes in a couple of shade options (plus a shimmery version); our testers trialled the 'fair to normal skin' shade. (One tester thought she had a sensitivity reaction.)

Testers say: 'Perfect texture to apply; light without being greasy; no discernible colour after one application, then built up a subtle light biscuity colour' • 'slightly fruity smell; gave a realistic tan, then faded evenly' • 'didn't leave a residue; built to healthy-looking natural colour' • 'liked the subtle shimmer; perfect for getting some colour on your skin before a holiday' • 'very realistic'.

tried & tested
leg tints

An absolute godsend, these, for that first, post-black-opaques day of summer when you want to wear a skirt – but your legs look like they've spent the winter under a stone. (A great alternative to fake tans, too, if you dislike that biscuity smell.)

L'Oréal Sublime Bronze One Day

 We admit we burst through our £10 'ceiling' for this. But – to paraphrase L'Oréal – it's because it's worth it. An innovative new formula, it contains pearl particles for a subtly luminous tint, which is more golden than most (they tend to have pinky undertones). The 'sunny-fragranced' gel stays in place – even if it rains – and won't budge till you remove with soap or shower gel.

Testers say: 'A fabulous alternative to self-tan because it's goof-proof – the smooth gel really did make my legs look like I'd been on vacation, and it's much less drying than some' • 'so easy to use and control; a rich bronze – just like my natural tan without going red first!' • 'easy to apply and it sank in quickly' • 'simply the best I've ever tried'.

> # *tip*
>
> **In an emergency, you can fake a sunkissed look with – yes – cold tea (just like they used to, in the war). Simply squeeze some used teabags, and stroke on to legs in smooth strokes. It does work, but it's a faff, so only for a real pastry-leg SOS.**

Sally Hansen Airbrush Legs

 'A unique spray-on make-up for legs' is how Sally Hansen describes this aerosol, in four shades, from Light Glow to Deep Glow, so you can match your skintone. The formula, they say, is designed to cover up spider veins, blemishes and freckles. We've featured this before, and it remains a classic – now much used on the catwalk at London Fashion Week.

Testers say: 'Very happy to use instead of fake tan; I liked the results – good colour for light coverage' • 'really natural colour' • 'useful for top-ups on holiday' • 'washed off easily with soap or shower gel' • 'can spray upside down for backs of legs' • 'good for wearing skirts in summer' • 'didn't smudge or rub off'.

 ### Solait Sexy Legs

Superdrug's option: a light gel texture dispensed from a flip-top cap, this has the merest whisper of

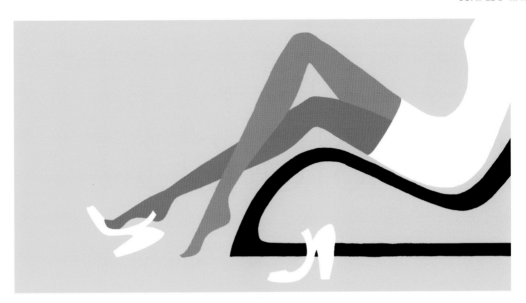

shimmer. Our testers had the lighter 'Golden' shade; 'Bronze' is for a deeper tan effect.

Testers say: 'I loved this: much more even finish than self-tan; it's instant and you can control the results' • 'went on like a moisturiser; gave a natural, pale golden glow you could build up for more colour' • 'I dressed almost straight away; colour still looked good and none had rubbed off by bedtime' • 'gave a healthy light glow to my uncooked-pork-sausage legs'.

Vie at Home Perfection

6.75/10 Are you ready to airbrush your legs? Basically, that's what you do

♥ *we love*

Very occasionally we join a panel, trial products and fill in forms like the rest of our testers. We both trialled the winning **L'Oréal Sublime Bronze One Day** product – and loved it so much it's now on our bathroom shelves.

with this can: zhoosh the product on, then give it a final blend with fingers – which some testers found tricky. (Again, this product just busts our price point – sorry.)

Referred to as 'invisible tights' by Vie at Home (who used to be Virgin Vie), it's based on face foundation technology and contains aloe vera gel, to moisturise skin. Just one shade.

Testers say: 'Top marks; like very thin foundation; didn't run down my legs; easy to blend in; light golden colour that looked as if I'd been tanning for a week' • 'dry in seconds; didn't rub off on clothes – best to do one leg at a time' • 'good for evening up my real tan – don't spray it near anything white!' • 'needed prepping – exfoliating, moisturising legs – but dried quickly, with no tacky film' • 'would be happy to use this but prefer a lotion/cream'.

tried & tested
spf15 moisturisers

These are a must, according to dermatologists we know – but as the excellent results prove, you really needn't break the bank to shield your skin against the ageing effects of UV light. (Trust us: prevention of wrinkles is much, much easier than cure.)

Skin Wisdom Restore & Replenish Perfecting Day Cream SPF15

8.12 / 10 Created by Ayurvedic beauty guru Bharti Vyas for Tesco, Skin Wisdom is an amazingly affordable range – with great results. This sub-brand in the Skin Wisdom collection was developed to nurture mature skin: a perfecting cream, blending wild yam, soy, rhodiola, red seaweed extract and skin-plumping hyaluronic acid, plus that so-vital SPF15.

Testers say: 'I loved this product and will buy it! It's white at first, but then disappears into the skin; make-up goes on very well after' • 'I didn't get shiny using this, which is a first for me – amazing!' • 'was impressed, as this is comparable with high-end products' • 'my face definitely looks better for it' • 'like the big pot: easy to get fingers in and out' • 'I got snobby about it coming from Tesco, but after using it, realised it could stand quite nicely beside more expensive products – and I would have more money to treat myself in other ways!' • 'very light, very effective, absorbed quickly, gorgeous smell – but I thought that 'holistic' would mean natural – and it's not, entirely'.

Skin Therapy Radiance Boost SPF15

8.05 / 10 Skin Therapy is Sainsbury's (very good) rival to Tesco's Skin Wisdom – here, a defending day formula which is formulated with

we love

pro-retinol (to improve skintone) and nourishing shea butter. Jo uses this and really does think the 'Radiance Boost' name is appropriate, as it seems to leave skin luminescent.

Testers say: 'Fab; skin feels smooth and moisturised, but not greasy; lovely base for make-up, too; no dry flaky skin around my nose, which I usually get' • 'good value, good product: I thought it would be too rich for my skin, but it sank in quickly' • 'felt light and dewy and make-up smoothed on easily' • 'product sank in beautifully; texture was smooth and felt luxuriously silky; some SPF face creams tend to be a little heavy and greasy – this was very light' • 'all-round good moisturiser'.

Eucerin Sensitive Skin Hydro-Protect SPF15 Normal To Dry Skin

7.61/10 Although the Eucerin range is just slightly above our usual price 'ceiling', we've included this for our many sensitive/dry-skinned readers, as tackling touchy skin is this range's claim to fame. (Sun-protective products are often major culprits when it comes to triggering sensitivity.) Eucerin claim 'three-in-one protection' with this, as it guards against environmental stress, UVA/UVB radiation and premature skin ageing, incorporating a plant-derived ingredient, alpha-glucosylrutin (which helps protect plants from damage), plus vitamin E. But testers emphasise that it is for drier skins.

Testers say: 'Good moisturiser; left no dry patches at all; felt as though I had a barrier on; left dewy moist effect – which I blotted before applying mineral powder foundation' • 'liked the fact this had vitamin E – very good for fighting free radicals!' • 'effective moisturiser; skin felt softer, smoother and comfortable on the cheeks, where I sometimes have small dry patches – gave a radiant, dewy, but quite shiny appearance' • 'colleague thought I looked dewy skinned; two people separately told me I looked glowing!' • 'a real find for my sensitive skin – I have trialled many products at different prices; I will definitely buy this'.

Botanics Skin Calming Cream for Sensitive and Dry Skin

7.55/10 Another product – as the name implies - for sensitive skins, from the successful Boots range which famously incorporates active plant extracts. Here, marshmallow is the key botanical, with its renowned soothing action, together with nourishing shea butter – and although the SPF15 isn't advertised in the product name, it is there in the jar.

Testers say: 'A good no-frills moisturiser which left skin nourished and soothed without flaring up any of my oilier patches; easy to get out of the pot'•'dew-silky effect, and if I was having a good skin day, I would happily leave the house with no make-up on; I was really impressed'•'it says to wear this morning and night, but I think it's a bit daft to wear an SPF in the dark'•'soaked in easily and made my face feel lovely and soft; looked dewy and really did plump up my skin; beautiful fragrance, like marshmallows – I could have eaten it – I was really impressed by this cream'•'a great budget buy'.

Healthspan Nurture Replenish Day Cream SPF15

 Healthspan Nurture is a mail-order only company, marketing supplements and affordable skincare. The Replenish range is aimed at more mature and post-menopausal complexions, 'to help feed back important oestrogen and collagen to the skin' (so they tell us), using plant oestrogens. (Healthspan Nurture take a two-way approach to beauty, so there is also a supplement in the range to support the age-defying efficacy of this product.)

Testers say: 'Nice creamy consistency; keeps my face from getting tight after cleansing'•'make-up went on well if I left 10-15 minutes after applying moisturiser'•'thick, luxurious cream; skin felt hydrated and supple'•'leaves skin soft, and slightly dewy but not greasy: make-up didn't slide off'•'left a lovely sheen; I used too much at first, but when I got amount right, it was lovely'• 'I would use this if my skin was very dry'•'loved this product – very effective; made skin moist and plump. A must-have'.

Bharti Vyas (Skin Wisdom creator) advises: 'Apply facial skincare to your neck and down to the breast bone. Moisturising these areas effectively will help prevent them giving away your biological age.' And remember, neck and chest are so perfectly angled to pick up sun damage…

Tinted moisturisers

We've always found that a touch of sun – in a tube – is a very good way to perk up a face fast. Very respectable results for these wash-off tinted moisturisers – you'd be surprised by some of the big names languishing behind these, in our chart. NB: if you have dry skin, you may need to apply a light moisturiser underneath, too.

 Skin Wisdom Instant Benefits Visibly Radiant Tinted Moisturiser

 Skin Wisdom – Bharti Vyas's range for Tesco – has lots of different sub-ranges within it: Instant Benefits covers the products targeted at all ages, designed to 'offer fast fixes for common skin complaints'. This very affordable tinted moisturiser put in a really great performance for the price: a suits-all-skintones shade which sinks in and softens to a radiant but not shiny finish.

Active ingredients include acerola cherry and vitamin C (for radiance), and moisturising honey (though it's not sticky). **Testers say:** 'Goes on really smoothly and is quite effective as a moisturiser, but my dry skin looked better if I "prepped" with a dab of my usual day cream first' • 'went on evenly and blended effortlessly into my skin; gave my skin some radiance' • 'looked dark in the tube but was so natural on my skin – just seemed to enhance it, rather than colour it; but didn't cover thread veins' • 'my skin looks better when I'm wearing this: nice to grab and go, to top up the post-holiday tan'.

Olay Complete Care Touch of Foundation

 Olay tell us they created this for 'the 83 per cent of women across the world who say they don't like to wear too much make-up every day'. It may be called 'Touch of Foundation' but actually, it's sheer and behaves like a tinted moisturiser (but some testers needed a moisturiser too). It has a 'light dosage' of Max Factor foundation pigments, and is

tip **If you don't want to spring for a tinted moisturiser, mix your favourite primer or moisturiser half and half with liquid foundation. (Remember that if either 'ingredient' has an SPF, you will only be getting half the protection.) The advantage is that you can customise the amount of cover you want – a touch more if you have broken veins, for instance, or less, if you want a sheerer finish.**

packed with 'Olay moisture' and vitamin E, for a fresh-faced look. **Testers say:** 'My skin felt moisturised and nourished day long; feels very light, applying it to skin, which looks fresher, brighter and not as congested; evened out skintone, but you need a concealer for any flaws' • 'so light people thought I was wearing nothing on my face' • 'good base for mineral powder foundation; dispenser was fine' • 'people said I looked well and healthy; the colour looked dark but was well suited to my skin, and no orangey tint' • 'easy to apply, evened out skintone, gave light coverage – heaven!'.

Vie At Home Sheer Perfection SPF15 Tinted Moisturiser

 As this tied with the Olay product above, we felt we should include it, as

it's only £1 more expensive, is also available in three shades (Light, Medium and Dark) and likewise features a useful SPF15 sunscreen. Vie At Home (formerly Virgin Vie) tell us this contains jojoba oil, to keep skin dewily radiant all day long. NB: we were sent the lightest shade. **Testers say:** 'I was very pleased with this: I can't wear foundation, as it is too thick and mineral make-up sinks into lines and, because of my dry skin, makes me look like a made-up corpse! This evened out my skintone so I looked and felt better – I am so pleased I have found something, finally' • 'easy to blend evenly after applying moisturiser; skin looked more radiant and only needed a little concealer round the nose; good packaging' • 'easy to blend; no patchiness; skin looked more glowy'.

tried & tested
facial suncare

We get so many anxious e-mails to www.beautybible.com asking us what women can do about lines and wrinkles – but the bottom line is that prevention is way, WAY more effective than cure – and the main line of prevention is to use a sunscreen. There aren't many shining stars in this category, but these three did tick most of the boxes for our testers. Our advice is still to wear a hat and wide-armed sunglasses, as well. And if you really want a bronzed face…fake it!

Neal's Yard Remedies Lemongrass Sun Spray SPF10

7.92/10 Organic soya, sesame and wheatgerm oils blend with skin-nourishing horse chestnut in this spritz-on sun protector, suited to both face and body, albeit with a relatively low SPF10. Some loved the lemongrass smell , others not – so best to sniff before buying.

Testers say: 'This worked surprisingly well initially, but wore off faster than my usual brand, what with sweat and travelling, so need to reapply often' • 'very pleasant fresh fragrance: was absorbed really quickly and felt nice on my skin' • 'my face looked freshly moisturised but there was no noticeable oiliness; my skin didn't react at all to the sun, with this;

I would use it on a daily basis for the easy application and moisturisation it gave' • 'liked the sheen it left on my skin'.

Garnier Ambre Solaire SPF30 Sheer Protect Hydrating Face Protection Cream

7.44/10 This hydrating formula features Garnier's photo-stable sun protection filters Mexoryl® XL and SL – which

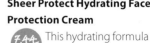

means it doesn't break down in sunlight (unlike many). It is designed to shield against premature ageing, and also brown spots. Suitable for sun-sensitive skins, the formula is non-sticky and non-greasy. (It just breaks through our £10 barrier – but we felt we should include it because facial suncare is such an important skincare category.)

Testers say: 'Loved this product: my face felt comfortable and healthy – I'll be using it all year, as it's great to find high protection that's so moisturising'•'leaves a summery pearlescent sheen on the skin'•'smells slightly of coconut and peaches and reminds me of sunny beaches and being on holiday'•'very effective: left dry parts feeling moisturised and didn't leave my T-zone shiny or greasy'•'I use Decléor, usually, which is great but expensive – and am pleased to find Ambre Solaire does the same thing!'

 Soleil Beauty Face Defence Matte Fluid Anti-Wrinkle SPF30

7.37/10 An extraordinarily low price for a product that incorporates anti-ageing

tip

It's so tempting to keep suncare from one season to the next, if you haven't used every last squeeze before the end of your holiday – but the strength of the SPF may diminish, over the winter months. What you can do – rather than waste it – is to use a facial product on your body next season: facial suncare generally has a higher SPF than body suncare, and faces need more protection than the rest of our skin. If you've got leftover body products, though, the bin beckons: it's too much of a gamble to get them out of the bathroom cupboard after six to nine months.

ingredients (it's enriched with blackberry leaf extract, among other constituents, to help reduce sun-induced breakdown of collagen). Like

the Garnier product, it sinks in fast and doesn't leave an oily film; this is also water-resistant and delivers 12-hour 'proven moisturisation' – although several testers found they needed a moisturiser as well. (The same formulation is also available at SPF50, though the increased benefit of this over SPF30 is very slight, according to experts.)

Testers say: 'Pleasantly surprised that the product was easily absorbed without my having to rub it in too much – the shade gave me a little bit of colour and took the edge off my paleness on a day when I was very tired'•'great under make-up, as it's a light product and gives a matt-ish finish'•'rubbed in very easily and left a nice glow; didn't feel too thick or claggy, as these products sometimes do'•'really liked the fragrance – fresh and not sickly'•'good pump dispenser – probably not suitable for your handbag, though'•'nice velvety texture and made skin soft and smooth, but wasn't deeply moisturising'•'I'll be using this instead of my usual product'•'no irritation or redness'•'very light compared to most sunscreens, especially those with an SPF30'.

tried & tested
body suncare

There's something here for everyone: high SPFs, medum SPFs, sun-protective lotions, oils – and a 'lightweight' product for anyone who doesn't like the heaviness of many sun products. All reasonable (or reasonable-ish) – and many outperforming a lot of much pricier options.

NB: a couple of the non-supermarket products featured here come in slightly above our £10 'ceiling'. Suncare is generally priced well above normal skincare. We hate to be conspiracy theorists about this, but could that be because brands know we're paranoid about sun damage – and we'll pay that bit extra? Hmmm.

 Soleil Beauty Light Hydrating Milk SPF30

 A very high score indeed for this product, which comes in a flip-top orange bottle, and features what Tesco (whose own-label range Soleil is) describe as 'skin-firming actives',

while it's also said to protect against age spots. It's water resistant, and delivers proven 12-hour moisturisation.

Testers say: 'Felt more like a moisturiser on my skin than a sun lotion – not at all greasy; disappeared when rubbed in (hardly needed any rubbing) and left a slight sheen; liked the botanicals among the synthetic ingredients' • 'very effective; skin felt really nourished and soft, as well as being protected: I would definitely buy this over my normal one' • 'love the fragrance; smells like holidays' • 'feels very light in comparison to other brands' • 'loved this on my skin – made it instantly smoother and radiant'.

Nivea Sun Light Feeling Sun Lotion SPF30

One reason people shy away from using sun products is their traditionally heavy and/or sticky texture, but this is airier than most, glides over skin as it's being applied – and sinks in fast.

Testers say: 'Nice, fresh moisturising cream that felt light and comfortable, didn't clump on hairs, and smoothed in easily; left a slight sheen, but no white marks – and no burning!' • 'I really look forward to using this: the smell is wonderful, and it is not at all greasy' • 'I am very impressed with this: it does exactly what it says on the bottle – felt lovely, cool and light, and no sticky coating; I would definitely buy it' • 'I will be switching to this from now on; my boyfriend is happy to use it, too, because it's not greasy, and the fragrance is very light'.

Malibu Dry Oil Spray SPF15

 Malibu recommend spritzing skin with this fast-drying, waterproof, non-

we love

greasy oil 30 minutes before heading for the sun. With a chemical UVA/UVB screen, it can be sprayed through the hair to protect the scalp. Good for men, who tend not to like rubbing sun cream into hairy chests.

Testers say: 'I was expecting it to be greasy, oily and sticky: it soaked in almost immediately – I am a total convert'•'as effective as more expensive sun preps; feel texture wouldn't block pores, so may help my sun allergy'•'smells of sun-drenched beaches and piña colada'•'this was moisturising but sank in immediately; no rubbing needed' •'no redness or burning'.

Garnier Ambre Solaire High SPF 30 Moisturising Protection Spray

7.5/10 Garnier's products used to be called just Ambre Solaire. Within the bafflingly large range, our testers particularly liked this 'Very High SPF30': the spray makes it easy to spritz hard-to-access areas, and the formula is non-greasy yet moisturising.

Testers say: 'Tried this on a very sunny day, near the equator, and it was perfect! No annoying scent, not oily, super easy to

---

---

apply and protected my skin totally'•'a good product that I will buy again: good moisturisation; disappeared quite quickly; better than my usual brand'•'skin felt soft after applying and looked slightly dewy; needed a little rubbing in, but not hugely more than my usual brand'•'packaging is easy to hold, and to spray out the right amount'•'this holds its own with my usual brands, based on price and UV protection; light and easily wearable'.

tip

A recent *Which?* report confirmed that the SPF which suncare delivers may not always match the figure on the bottle. We recommend reapplying frequently, to keep the SPF 'topped up'. Once is not enough...

Sainsbury's Sun Protect Spray SPF15

7.1/10 A very lightweight and fresh-scented formulation which features antioxidant vitamin E and other ingredients for longlasting skin hydration. Water-resistant, too.

Testers say: 'Very effective and pleasant to use, though took a bit of rubbing in'•'light feeling, but moisturising'•'lotion disappeared almost immediately, leaving skin soft'•'a really nice smooth feel; very pleasing – nice fresh smell: a pleasure to use'•'pretty effective: I also used it on my face, which it says you can in the very small print! More of an emulsion, and needs some rubbing in, but that didn't take long'•'fantastic value for money; good-quality packaging, and application was great – it melted into the skin and was easily absorbed; gave a nice sheen without being greasy'.

tried & tested
after-suns

We're impressed. The high street and drugstore brands featured here actually scored way higher than some of the really pricy options (one was over £100!) that we trialled at the same time. We say: less money on suncare = more money for ice cream!

Soleil Beauty Tan Accelerating Aftersun Lotion

 Tesco promise 'premium sun protection at great Tesco prices', and this winning entry taps into the trend for 'tan-accelerating' products. Its key ingredient: a 'bio-complex' called Phototan®, alongside shea butter and soothing allantoin, plus an antioxidant complex to protect skin. Tesco also tell us it delivers 12-hour hydration.

Testers say: 'Very easy to apply; sank in easily; pleasant smell of shea butter; felt moisturising and refreshing and my skin was soft and smooth' • 'liked that the packaging can be recycled' • 'really lovely cooling effect; relieved mild tightness; really moisturising – did everything it claimed. I'd definitely buy it' • 'lovely, fresh, fruity summertime aroma' • 'calmed down my pink skin; my husband now uses this every night for its cooling, redness-reducing and super-moisturising effects'.

Piz Buin After Sun Tan Prolonger Lotion

 A big, fat, skin-soothing tub of cream, which – like the entry above – contains an ingredient to boost the skin's own natural melanin production and thus preserve your tan for up to two weeks after you're back home. (They call it 'Tanimel', and it comes from a natural root plant extract, *Ononis spinosa*). This, Piz Buin tell us, quenches skin thirst for 24 hours.

Testers say: 'Left my legs softer, smoother and with a faint glow – a bit like using a gradual tanner; like the thick, cooling cream, but would decant into a smaller pot for transporting' • 'very smooth, and my body felt velvety to the touch after – made my fake tan look more natural!' • 'very hydrating, so keeps your tan longer' • 'very light in texture, with a floral body-lotion smell'.

Nivea Sun Moisturising After Sun Lotion

 A multiple award-winning entry (and not just from us!), this sinks-in-fast intensive moisturising formulation from one of the ultimate classic skincare brands offers vitamin E (to help fight premature ageing), and is enriched with aloe vera and skin-nurturing avocado oil.

Testers say: 'Fantastic product – which relieved my bad sunburn immediately; this will have a place in my beach bag for ever!' • 'lovely fragrance made it a pleasure to use; sank in fairly quickly, leaving skin soft, smooth – pleasant to "wear", rather than tight and stretched' • 'such a lovely lotion – leaves the skin soft and silky; immediate cooling sensation that always relieves sunburn instantly; I enjoy the smell, the cooling and moisturising – it never fails me'.

Garnier Ambre Solaire After Sun Hydrating Tan Maintainer

 Garnier's range scored incredibly well across the board with our tester panels – they have winning facial and body suncare entries, too – and

tip

Plenty of after-suns now contain cooling ingredients – but when the going gets hot, a free option is to keep a spray bottle of water in the fridge and spritz yourself. As the water evaporates, you'll cool right down. (You can also keep your after-sun in the fridge if you're staycationing at home.) And our long-term favourite is pure aloe gel, either straight from a leaf (simply snap and squeeze) or a tube of organic aloe vera from any health store.

among the summer sun treats our testers ranked highly is this high-tech moisturiser, which is also designed to prolong your tan's life, enriched with cactus extract to soothe and nourish.

Testers say: 'Immediately felt my skin cool down – very refreshing' • 'smells fresh and natural, with a scent of aloe vera' • 'safely portable screw-top tube' • 'really smooth application – melted right in, even on wet skin' • 'like the subtle self-tanning effect – helps with that "just been on holiday" look' • 'I'd use this product during the winter to add some colour and life to my pale skin'.

Soltan Aftersun Gel

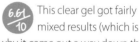 This clear gel got fairly mixed results (which is why it came out a way down the list), but some testers really enjoyed the extra-cooling formulation, which features aloe vera to soothe and moisturise effectively. The fact that it can be used on faces and bodies also endeared it to some testers.

Testers say: 'This felt cool to touch, and would be soothing for sunburn; no sticky residue; very moisturising and skin softening' • 'easy portable packaging; attractive fresh scent and slight cooling sensation' • 'I think this product would be useful for children' • 'slightly gooey, but not sticky at all; my skin felt very soft after use; very cooling and fresh'.

tried & tested
tweezers

Lordy, we've used some dreadful cheap tweezers in our day – not fit for purpose, with zero grip. These, by contrast, are easy-tweezy winners: high-quality tools at great prices, for instant brow-'zing'.

Revlon Diamond Grip Tweezers

7.87/10 Revlon's accessories range is a bestseller, Stateside, and includes these: the tips of the white-enamelled tweezers are coated with real diamond particles for maximum gripping power of even the shortest, finest hairs. They have a little black sleeve to slip over the end for protection.

Testers say: 'Easy enough to hold – very comfortable, nice length and fit neatly in the hand; grip even the shortest hairs well' •'like the little pouch, though it was a bit boring being black; would prefer a pattern'•'quite comfy; just sharp enough; easy to select individual hairs to pluck, and picked out a lot of regrowth/short hairs with ease, from my thick brows – I would buy'•'a person with thick hairs will find them a godsend'•'very impressed with appearance and little protective pouch' •'super-easy to use; really good for getting all the hairs – like the angled tip, and nice spring between the prongs'•'plastic handle made it much easier to hold the tweezers and plucking much more accurate – I feel very confident using them, better than my own ones: I have recommended them to friends'.

♡ we love

Jo jealously guards her Revlon Diamond Grip Tweezers from goddaughters/granddaughters, who are plucking obsessed – and also loves the Revlon 10 x Magnifeye Tweezing Mirror, in the same accessories collection, which reveals even the teensiest stray hairs. (It's not wise to shape your whole brow using a magnifying mirror, though, as you need to get an overview of the brow shape, but good for a final clean-up.) Sarah only likes slant-edged ones, preferably Tweezerman – she can never make the pointy ones pick up hairs!

M&S Autograph Slanted Tweezers

7.2/10 Something a bit different: these slant-tweezers have a built-in blue LED light, which you click on when you want extra illumination while you pluck, and come with a teensy mirror in a plastic sleeve. There's a black pochette to keep the lot in (and – see our TIP – we can't recommend highly enough that you do).

Testers say: 'These grasped hairs very well; worked well on most hairs, except the very tiniest; my existing tweezers were quite expensive but vicious – I found it difficult to pluck hairs without getting bits of skin, too; these were just right' • 'nothing wrong with these at all – well made, well presented and more than adequate for purpose – but they don't compare with my slightly more expensive Tweezerman Slant Tip tweezers' • 'lovely packaging – the little holder with magnetic clip was fantastic for transporting them around easily' • 'comfortable in the hand and quite springy, I liked the slanted design and the pouch' • 'excellent tweezers that coped with my very fine brow hairs' • 'I thought tweezers were tweezers – but these were great tweezers!'.

tip

If your tweezers come with a sleeve or protective wallet, invest in the extra second to put the sleeve back on – every single time. The minute that tweezers are even slightly bent, they lose their grip and it's 'over and out'. So, ideally, keep at home, in the bathroom cabinet, in their sleeve (or wrapped in a hankie, if no sleeve is provided). Then they're on hand for regular plucking – preferably by the light of a window – or in a (stationary) car mirror.

e.l.f. Perfect Tweezers

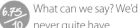 What can we say? We'd never quite have believed that a pair of tweezers which costs less than two quid could possibly rival some pricier versions (though Tweezerman fans remain devoted), but these – 'ergonomically designed for easy and accurate tweezing' – ones are said to be professional quality, and our testers were (mostly) happy, especially with the bargain basement price-tag. Like all tweezers, they'll benefit from being kept in a safe place (see TIP).

Testers say: 'Top marks. They work perfectly: sharp enough but not too sharp. Fantastic – they grabbed the right hair every time' • 'very comfortable and easy to use; easy to hold, and nice ends that were just right to work with; I have fine blonde hairs, so was surprised at how easily they plucked them; almost as good as my expensive set. Amazing price for the quality; being so affordable lets me have a pair in the bathroom as well as in my make-up case and handbag' • 'fit well into hand and easy to use; strong grip, so you need to be quite firm; terrier-like grip on short or fine hairs; brilliant for putting on false eyelashes, as they hold on to the lash firmly, so you can glue them and position with ease' • 'fairly comfortable, but quite heavy; great style; not very good for grabbing single hairs, but would be great for tidying up bikini line'.

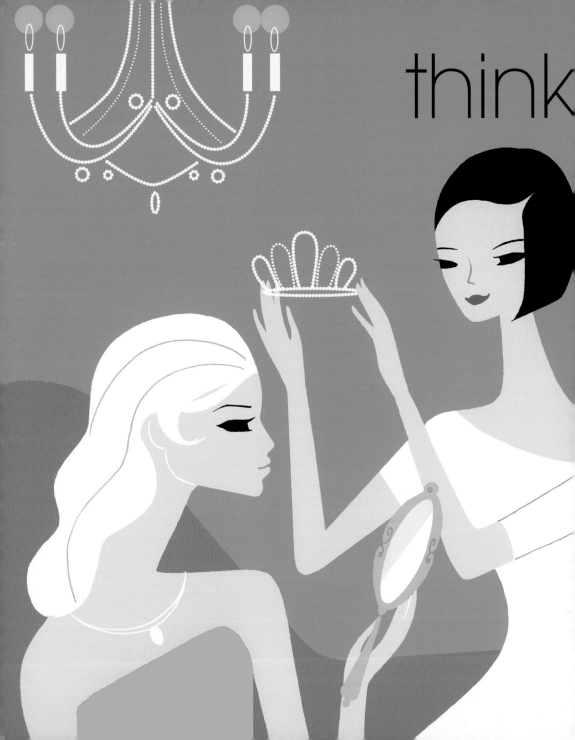

think

ourself lovely

Hands up now: anyone not want to look gorgeous? And we all can, according to our favourite gorgeousness guru, Gok Wan, presenter of TV makeover shows: 'The key is to develop confidence – just think: I am GORGEOUS!'

First, ask your best friend to play a little game: you tell her three features about her face that are pretty, then she tells you. Be imaginative: laughing eyes, cute freckles, pretty ear lobes, smooth forehead, delicious hairline…get it?

Then list three about your bodies: say, swan neck, satiny décolletage, elegant back, neat ankles.

Remember: you're only allowed to say full-on nice, loving words. And the rule is that you have to accept compliments graciously – after all, you're worth it…

Set up a 'mirror moment': shut the door, strip off and take a long look. Remember: it will only look really bad once. Keep looking and the iffy bits (boobs, bum, tum, thighs, for most women) won't be so bad. Now look at the good bits you've identified – and work on those.

Improve your posture: you can 'lose' five pounds in ten seconds. So – pull up your body from your ankles, knees, up your spine to the crown of your head, let your shoulders drop back and your bosom float up, lift your eyes and look ahead and away.

Our tip: join a yoga class – it's the quickest way to mind and body grace. (For short sequences for specific purposes, such as posture, sleep, PMS, visit www.hannahlovegrove.com – the website of one of our fave Iyengar yoga teachers.)

Finally: remember the adage – glamour is ten per cent what you look like and 90 per cent what other people think you do. Looking lovely is never about being perfect – no one is, not even supermodels. As Gok says: 'Stop judging, start loving.' Love yourself, be loving, accept love – and, with a titchy bit of upkeep, you'll all be princesses! It's that simple.

And what do princesses wear?

Tiaras, of course. For reasons we simply can't remember, a group of us (all in the beauty world) started to have 'tiara teas' for birthdays. We wear our sparkly tiaras at these (a SuperSteal from an accessory shop in North London) and have also been known to put them on to do the hoovering – or just because it's a grey day. Try it!

directory

All product names and prices were correct at the time of going to press. But, just in case anything changes, this list is also on our website, www.beautybible.com, and we'll update it regularly. (Look for the BEAUTY STEALS button in the left-hand margin.) In addition, do visit the site and check out our INSIDER DISCOUNTS button (at the top of the page), where you can take advantage of exclusive beautybible.com discounts on hundreds of brands – making every beauty purchase more steal-like!

A'kin
www.victoriahealth.com

Alberto Balsam
Available nationwide

Alida
01707 292938, www.alida.co.uk

Andrew Collinge
Available nationwide
www.andrewcollinge.com

Aromatherapy Associates
020 8569 7030,
www.aromatherapyassociates.com

Aveeno
0845 601 5791, www.aveeno.co.uk

Avon
0845 601 4040, www.avonshop.co.uk

Badger Balms
01827 280 080,
www.beautynaturals.co.uk

Balance Me
www.balanceme.co.uk

Balm Balm
www.balmbalm.com

Barbara Daly
0800 505 555.
Available from Tesco nationwide
www.tesco.com

Beautifully Delicious
0845 070 8090, www.boots.com
Available in Boots, Sainsbury's and
Morrison's, UK

Beauty Bible Lip Balm
www.victoriahealth.com

Bioré
0845 070 8090, www.boots.com

The Body Shop
01903 844 554, www.thebodyshop.co.uk

Boots
0845 070 8090, www.boots.com

Botanics
0845 070 8090, www.boots.com

Bourjois
0800 269 836, www.bourjois.co.uk

Burt's Bees
0845 270 3635, www.iloveburt.com

Carnation Footcare
0121 544 7117,
www.carnationfootcare.co.uk

Champneys
0800 636 262, www.champneys.co.uk

Clinique
0870 034 2666, www.clinique.co.uk

Collection 2000
01695 727317,
www.collection2000.co.uk

Corn Silk
www.amazon.co.uk

Crabtree & Evelyn
01443 445566, www.crabtree-evelyn.co.uk

Cutex
Available nationwide

d:fi
www.hqhair.com   www.slapiton.tv

Dove
0800 085 1548, www.boots.com
Available nationwide

Daniel Galvin Junior
01795 581 151, www.danielgalvinjnr.co.uk

**Dr Bronner's range of Organic Castile
Liquid Soaps**
0845 072 5825, www.pureskincare.co.uk

Dr Organic Bioactive Skincare
0870 606 6606,
www.hollandandbarrett.com

EcoTools
01344 878 180.
Available from Tesco & Superdrug stores
nationwide.

Elegant Touch
www.eleganttouch.co.uk

e.l.f. Healthy Glow Bronzing Powder
0845 678 8818, www.eyeslipsface.co.uk

Elle Macpherson
www.boots.com

Elvive
Available nationwide

Essential Care
01638 716 593, www.essential-care.co.uk

Eucerin
0845 644 8556, www.eucerin.co.uk

Faith in Nature
0161 724 4016, www.faithinnature.co.uk

FCUK
www.boots.com

Free Zone
(Selected Sainsbury's) 0800 636 262

Garnier
Available nationwide, www.garnier.co.uk

Good Works
0845 070 8090, www.boots.com
Available from Boots stores nationwide

GOSH
0800 096 1055, www.superdrug.com

Green People
01403 740 350, www.greenpeople.co.uk

Healthspan Nurture
0800 072 9510,
www.healthspan.co.uk/

Herbal Essences
Available nationwide

James Brown
www.boots.com. From Boots stores
nationwide

Jason
0845 072 5825. Available from health and
natural food stores nationwide

Jergens
www.boots.com
At Boots stores nationwide

John Frieda
020 7851 9800, www.johnfrieda.com

John Masters
www.victoriahealth.com

Kiehl's
www.spacenk.com

Korres
020 7581 6455, www.korres.com

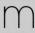

Lavera
01557 870567, www.lavera.co.uk

Lee Stafford
0870 351 8004, www.leestafford.com

Lipcote
www.lipcote.com

Liz Earle Naturally Active Skincare
01983 813913, www.lizearle.com

L'Oréal
www.lorealparis.co.uk
Available nationwide

Louise Galvin Natural Locks
www.louisegalvin.com

M.A.C. Cosmetics
0870 0342676, www.maccosmetics.com

Malibu
01923 289 470, www.malibusun.com

Marks & Spencer
0845 302 1234, www.marksandspencer.com

Mavala
01732 459 412, www.mavala.co.uk

Max Factor
www.maxfactor.co.uk

Maybelline
0845 399 0304, www.maybelline.co.uk

Me Me Me
0800 096 1055, www.superdrug.com

Ms. Pedicure
0845 070 8090. Available from Boots stores
nationwide

myface.cosmetics
www.boots.com
Available from Boots stores nationwide

Neal's Yard Remedies
0845 262 3145, www.nealsyardremedies.com

Nivea
0845 644 8556, www.nivea.co.uk

Neutrogena
0845 601 5789, www.neutrogenauk.co.uk

No 7
0845 070 8090, www.boots.com

Olay
0800 085 0367, www.olay.co.uk

OPI
01923 240 010, www.lenawhite.co.uk

Organic Bloom by Skin Blossom
05600 533 049, www.lovelula.com

Organic Blue
0208 952 2020, www.organicblue.com

Organic Surge
01955 606 061, www.organicsurge.com

Origins
0800 074 6905, www.origins.co.uk

Palladio Cosmetics
0845 094 0400, www.beautynaturals.com

Palmer's
Available from Boots, Superdrug and leading
supermarkets. www.chemistdirect.com

Papier Poudre
020 3260 3750, www.papierpoudre.co.uk

Perfect 10
www.originaladditions.com

Piz Buin
www.boots.com
From Boots stores nationwide

Pond's
0800 591720

Prestige
0845 070 8090, www.boots.com

Purely Skincare
www.purelyskincare.co.uk

r

Raw Gaia
01273 311476, www.rawgaia.com

Raw Minerals
www.rawbeauty.com

Red by Kiss
0845 070 8090, www.boots.com

Revlon
0800 085 2716, www.revlon.com

Rimmel
www.rimmellondon.com
Available from Boots and Superdrug stores
nationwide

Rose & Co
01827 280 080,
www.rose-apothecary.co.uk

S

Sainsbury's Active Naturals
0800 636 262, www.sainsburys.co.uk

Sally Hansen
www.sallyhansen.co.uk
At Boots stores nationwide

Samy
www.superdrug.com

The Sanctuary
www.boots.com
Available at Boots stores nationwide

Santé
0870 199 7838,
www.santecosmetics.co.uk

17
0845 070 8090, www.boots.com

Shockwaves
Available nationwide

Simple
0121 712 6523, www.simple.co.uk

Skinvitals
01622 859 898.
Available from Debenhams stores
nationwide

Sleek MakeUP
0800 096 1055, www.superdrug.com
Available from Superdrug stores nationwide

**Smudgees Eye Make-Up Smudge
Removers**
www.victoriahealth.com

Soap & Glory
0845 070 8090, www.boots.com

Solait
0800 096 1055, www.superdrug.com

Soleil Beauty
0800 505 555 www.tesco.com
Available from Tesco stores nationwide

Soltan
0845 070 8090, www.boots.com

Skin Therapy
0800 636 262.
Available from Sainsbury's stores
nationwide

Skin Wisdom
0800 505 555. Available from Tesco stores
nationwide

Superdrug
0800 096 1055, www.superdrug.com

This Works
0845 230 0499, www.thisworks.com

Time Delay
0845 070 8090, www.boots.com

Tisserand
01273 325 666, www.tisserand.com

Tommyguns
0845 688 0188, www.boots.com
From Boots stores nationwide

Toni & Guy
020 7440 6660, www.toniandguy.com

Treacle Moon
0800 505 555, www.treaclemoon.net
Available from Tesco stores nationwide

Tresemmé
0845 070 8090, www.tresemme.co.uk

Tri-Aktiline
0845 070 8090, www.boots.com

Tweezerman
www.HQhair.com

2True
0800 096 1055, www.superdrug.com

u

UMI
0800 188 884. At Waitrose stores
www.waitrose.com

v

Valerie Beverly Hills
www.victoriahealth.com

Vaseline
0800 085 1548. Available nationwide

Vie at Home
0845 300 8022, www.vieathome.com

W

Waitrose
0800 188 884, www.waitrose.com

Weleda
0115 944 8222, www.weleda.co.uk

Wella
01256 490 690. Available from
Wella Professional salons

W7
01753 639 137, www.magicmakeup.com

y

Yes to Carrots
www.victoriahealth.com

index

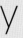

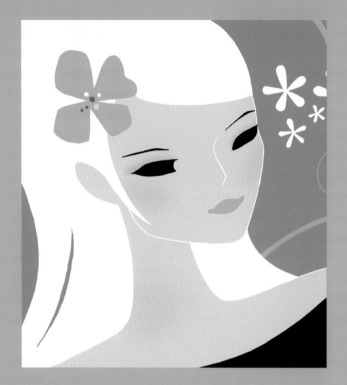

Sarah Stacey is an award-winning beauty and health journalist, and currently Health Editor of the *Mail on Sunday YOU* magazine. She has written for many leading newspapers and magazines in the UK and abroad. In 1994, she was elected the first Honorary Chair of the Guild of Health Writers UK and in 1996 was co-founder of the food labelling campaign, FLAG. She lives in west Dorset, near Lyme Regis, with a loyal and ancient Burmese cat and five large horses.

Josephine Fairley is a Contributing Editor to the *Mail on Sunday YOU* magazine, writing on beauty and organic living. She contributes to a wide range of publications including Red, Sainsbury's Magazine and the forthcoming National Geographic Green. A founding partner of Green & Black's Organic Chocolate, she now also runs Judges Bakery, an organic artisan bakery and food store, and recently opened The Wellington Centre, an 11-room boutique wellbeing centre; both are in Hastings, East Sussex.

We dedicate this book to Gill Sinclair — simply the best

Acknowledgements

Huge thanks to everyone involved in the mammoth production of this little tome. Without all of you, no book. We are truly grateful.

We'd like to start by thanking the Beauty Bible testers for their in-depth reporting (which sometimes had us in hysterics), and to the brands who continue generously to supply the products for those testers to put through their paces – making this the biggest-ever independent consumer test of beauty products on the planet.

To **Jessie Lawrence**, our Tried & Tested Co-ordinator, who put in more hours than we can bear to think at the screenface, and never lost her cool.

To the 'beauty elves' who toiled in the beauty dungeon: **Sacha Burrows**, **Lily de Kirkeriest** and most especially **Amy Eason**, our www.beautybible.com assistant, who sent out 24,000 products in the space of nine months. (No wonder she once came to work bleary-eyed, explaining: 'I dreamed of dancing beauty products, last night.') And to **David Edmunds**, who lugged tons of boxes and sacks down to and up from the dungeon.

To our much-loved agent **Kay McCauley**, as ever. And to the publishing team: **Kyle Cathie**, **Julia Barder**, **Sophie Allen** and **Victoria Scales**.

To our super-talented, super-nice creative team: designer **Jenny Semple** and illustrator **Orlando Hoetzel**. Also to unflappable copy editor **Simon Canney** and eagle-eyed proofreader **Liz Murray**.

To our webmaster **Ben Lovegrove**, the chap we totally can't do without – even though we drive him nuts.

And, lastly, to **Sue Peart**, **Catherine Fenton** and **Rosalind Lowe**, our colleagues at *YOU* magazine, for their unending support and niceness.

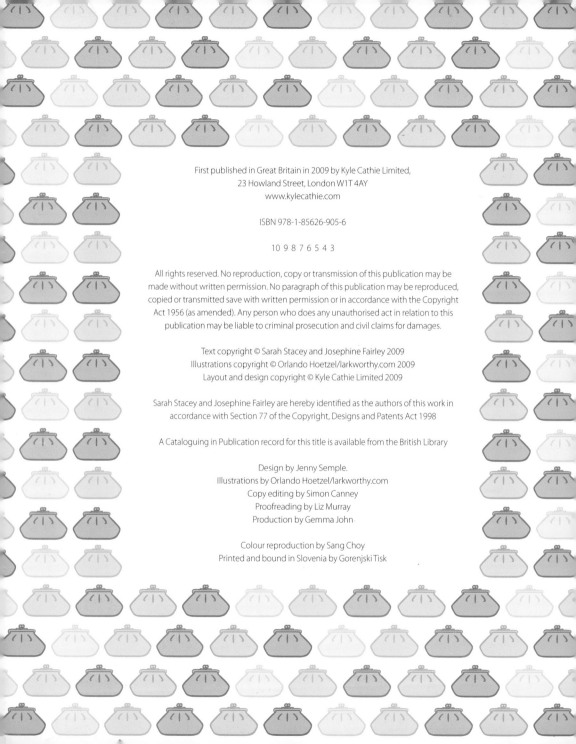

First published in Great Britain in 2009 by Kyle Cathie Limited,
23 Howland Street, London W1T 4AY
www.kylecathie.com

ISBN 978-1-85626-905-6

10 9 8 7 6 5 4 3

A Cataloguing in Publication record for this title is available from the British Library

Design by Jenny Semple.
Illustrations by Orlando Hoetzel/larkworthy.com
Copy editing by Simon Canney
Proofreading by Liz Murray
Production by Gemma John

Colour reproduction by Sang Choy
Printed and bound in Slovenia by Gorenjski Tisk